Community Ethics and
Health Care Research

Health and Nursing Studies for
Diploma and Undergraduate Students

Community Ethics
and
Health Care Research

Edited by

C Henry and G Pashley

Quay Books Division, Mark Allen Publishing Limited
Jesses Farm, Snow Hill, Dinton
Nr Salisbury, Wilts, SP3 5HN

British Library Cataloguing in Publication Data
A catalogue record for this book is available from the British Library

ISBN 1-85642-086-8
© 1995 Henry C and Pashley G

Printed in the UK by Biddles, Guildford.

Contents

List of Contributors

*Acknowledgement and thanks go to **Cathy Cookson**. Cathy has acted as Technical Editor on various books and publications for the present editors and shown always, great patience and kindness regarding our different grammatical styles!*

Christine Henry *has a professional background in Health, Psychology and Education. Her academic development at post graduate and doctorate level is in the areas of Philosophy, Ethics and Psychology specifically related to the Professional Fields of Education, Health, Research and Management. She is currently Professor of Applied Ethics, University of Central Lancashire. In 1992, she acted as research co-ordinator for the first Ethics and Values Audit in the UK.*

Glenys Pashley *has a background in Health, Psychology, Philosophy, Management and Research. She has a Masters Degree in Business Administration as well as one in Psychology and Education. She was involved in the first research based Ethics and Values Audit in the UK, carried out in the Centre for Professional Ethics at the University of Central Lancashire. She is currently a Senior Lecturer in Management and Social Work at the University of Central Lancashire.*

Laurie Wood *has recently completed her doctorate in Management and Organisational Studies, related to the Health Service Structure. She currently lectures in Management Theory at Salford University.*

Julie Apps *has a background in Nurse Education, Psychology and Ethics. She is currently studying for a PhD in Ethics and Psychology and is a Nurse Tutor in Manchester. She has published a significant number of articles in the health field.*

Mags Yeomans *has a background in Nursing and Education. She has also worked for the VSO, taught in schools and in Further Education, as well as being a Nurse Tutor. She has recently completed a Midwifery qualification and is currently working as a Midwife in Halifax.*

Kevin Kendrick *has a background in Nursing and Ethics. He is studying for his PhD in Ethics. He has published extensively in Nursing Ethics and is currently a Senior Lecturer in Ethics and Applied Philosophy at John Moore's University, Liverpool.*

Norman Fryer *has a background in Midwifery, Nursing and Health Care Management. She has recently completed her Masters in Health Ethics and is currently a Senior Lecturer in Midwifery and Ethics, and Co-ordinator for Research in the Department of Midwifery, University of Central Lancashire.*

June Davidson *has a background in Nursing, Health and Education. Her academic development at Masters level is within Education, Research and Nursing. She is currently Nurse Manager in the College of Health Studies, Northumbria University, Newcastle-upon-Tyne.*

Jeannie Siddique *has a background in Midwifery, Nursing and Education. She is currently studying for her MPhil/PhD. She is Senior Lecturer in Midwifery Studies and Course Leader for the BSc Professional Studies, University of Central Lancashire.*

Janine Drew *has a professional background in the diverse areas of Administration. Her academic interests are in English, Applied Ethics and Management Practice. She is currently studying for her PhD in Ethics and Management. She was a member of the research team for the first Ethics Audit carried out in the UK and is Principal Administrator at the University of Central Lancashire.*

Preface

Christine Henry and Glenys Pashley

An organisation, whether a hospital, a college, a university or even a company can be viewed from an 'other regarding caring perspective' as a community. The debate and questions raised throughout this text are hopefully held within the parameters of the term 'community' and hence the title of the text *Community Ethics and Health Care Research*.

This is the fourth volume in the series combining and expanding upon ethical and research areas. The text takes a rather different approach in its structure and content to that of the the first three introductory books. First, it is important to emphasise a more in-depth analysis and debate on major issues of professional ethics generally, and specifically, aspects of research itself. Second, it seems appropriate to prioritise concerns for the practitioner within times of rapid educational change. The text is divided into two major sections. One section deals with professional ethics, management and research issues and the other debates major aspects of applied research related to health and social care.

Undergraduates, postgraduate students and teachers will find this volume useful as a reference and teaching aid rather than as an introductory text. However, the book stands as a complete text, whilst at the same time complementing the other volumes.

New in this volume are areas concerned with detailed research issues which are not only relevant for health care practitioners but for other related professionals within the social and humanity domains. Issues of ethical debate involving professional ethics within education and health, raise questions of interest for management of care. Related epistemological concepts within applied science and psychology concerned with health and nursing practice are also examined.

A recurrent theme is the universalizable moral principle of 'respect for persons' that clearly is central to both health and social care. However, each chapter can be viewed separately, dealing with particular ethical issues relevant to professional practice, whether it is within nursing, health, medicine, social, education or research practice.

Section 1
Professional ethical perspectives
Prior to research

1 Professional ethics
Health, nursing, education and research
Christine Henry

'To see a World in a Grain of Sand/
And Heaven in a Wild Flower/
Hold Infinity in the palm of your hand/
And Eternity in an hour...........William Blake (1754–1827)

Being a professional

The word 'profession' has an historical origin within the religious community (Wilcox, 1992). To 'profess' means that members within a community profess vows. This not only emphasises membership but involves a commitment to a 'mission' for the community to follow 'rules of caring'. There are sociologically derived origins of being a professional. According to Evans (1991) roles are given, assigned or chosen and professionals undergo a socialisation process, learning the norms, conduct and those expectations of the chosen profession. The problem arises that a professional is often locked into this rigidly defined role and may adhere to a script defined by someone else. Within nursing, the doctor has been viewed as director of the script. The nurse may be other directed rather than inner directed (Evans, 1991). In this way, role prescriptions define what we are obligated to do to provide a service to society. According to Evans, the professional ethic that governs professional roles reinforces 'the way things are'. The professional may appeal to the professional ethic as a guide for action but the rules may not be relevant when she steps out of this role. As a member of the community, she must fall back upon the prescriptions of morality. In this sense, a sociological perspective, although shaping professional roles, can, on its own, inhibit the way we think and conceive of what we mean by being a professional.

Any organisation, through its management, will set goals and norms but this may not encourage moral behaviour.

In relation to 'being a professional', the structure and process within, and the pressures and demands from without, will influence individual integrity. If there is evidence of a slight change away from custom within an organisation, as a process of emancipating one's self as a professional, it may transform life for better or worse. There are some useful examples of this in major classical and modern literature, where authors have depicted characters in whom these changes from a professional sociological role result in the loss of individual integrity. Consequences of this are evident in the book *One Flew Over the Cuckoo's Nest*. The professional, i.e. the nurse, rigidly adheres to the sociological and organisational norms, juxtaposed with the emancipation, sometimes in extreme, of the patient under her care. Similar conflicts and emergent changes regarding roles and norms, with underpinning values, are evident in other works of literature, such as George Orwell's *Animal Farm*. There is increasing evidence available that supports the idea that ethics and values can be taught through the selective use of literature and, furthermore, highlights how values are, to some extent, socially constructed.

Midgley (1991) remarks that applied ethics and morality relate to the overlap of values amongst a variety of professions. Theory and practice are not distinctively separate. Practical ethics involve what we do, and how we behave, based upon the activity of making informed decisions from a professional standpoint.

> *"What does Crustomoney Proseed cake mean?" said Pooh.*
> *"For I am a Bear of Very Little Brain and long words bother me."*
> *"It means things to do."*
>
> *(Milne, 1926).*

Professional ethics

Factual belief and changes in laws of physics can occur rapidly and may be removed from ordinary life. Midgley remarks that moral rules are central to social and public life and the moral laws of society are of more immediate concern than the laws of physics. And, according to Midgley (1991b), the character of, perhaps, an engineer is not usually as important to his/her clients as that of a doctor, nurse or teacher. The personal impact is important and **valued** in face to face meetings.

Often, when we express strong feelings about a particular professional issue, it invokes criticism from others, indicating that we are being subjective or emotional. However, it is important to remember that feelings are part of being human and feeling strongly about something does not mean that there is an absence of thought. Whilst reason and informed judgment are crucial before taking action, imagination, creativity and feelings are equally a part of reflective thought and influence the way we 'practise what we preach'.

Morality refers to human conduct and values, whereas ethics refers to the study of these. 'Common-sense' dictates the two terms are interchangeable. If we avoid asking the metaphysical question, 'What is common-sense?' thus taking a practical view, common-sense can mean our perceptions, personal values, moral laws and our experience.

A code of conduct or practice can be viewed as guidelines that underpin statements of intent, sometimes referred to as mission statements or charters, e.g. *The Patient's Charter*. Operationalising a charter can be achieved through the professional's code of conduct or practice. A professional code of conduct will be reflected through action. However, both statements of intent, i.e. mission statements or charters and codes of conduct or practice will evolve from and are founded upon professional ethics, even though they, on their own, will not solve a moral dilemma.

Morals may be perceived as prescriptions or rules to guide our day to day human actions and behaviour, whereas ethics may be perceived as a set of analytical and descriptive tools. Ethics can be seen as a process to help identify right conduct and determine appropriate behaviour of the person. Morality is what we ideally aim for and ethics is a process that has a theoretical reflective and normative element that helps to achieve the aim. (Applied ethics is sometimes used interchangeably to mean normative or applied ethics. Professional ethics is also applied ethics).

Professional ethics can be a system of moral rules which prescribe the moral conduct of professionals. However, can we legitimately distinguish professional ethics from ordinary morality?

Evans remarks that a distinction can be made, in that ordinary morality derives moral principles which hold that rights and interests of all persons are equally worth protecting, but professional ethics may be seen as a set of rules, codes or specific conduct formulated, operated and enforced by the profession. The shared universal rule applicable to ordinary morality and to professional ethics is 'respect for persons'. Ethics can be further perceived as not only a process or tool but as the **outcome** of analytical and moral enquiry.

The process of professional ethics involves reflective investigation that weighs up alternatives, takes account of legal issues, feelings, mores and norms, personal values, perceptions and experience, but undertaking what we mean by professional ethics is, simply, to say there is a set of identified rules of conduct foundational upon the discipline of ethics. Furthermore, professional ethics is embodied in the 'ought of human conduct', striving for an ideal within the private and professional domains. There is central concern for practical issues that will usually result in action of some kind.

Professional autonomy

The term autonomy generally relates to the ethical principles of liberty and freedom of choice, being able to make informed decisions and to act in accordance with those decisions. In other words, to be self-determined. Thus personal autonomy is clearly being responsible, capable of independent judgements without being constrained by another person's action. Furthermore, ideally, personal autonomy means not having identifiable controlling mechanisms operating from either social, psychological or physical factors. However, personal autonomy is impossible. To take an example from everyday life, from a common-sense point of view, it is well known that any kind of emotional, psychological, social or physical disturbance will influence abilities. Simply having a common cold will impair judgement, as will being in a situation which is emotionally or psychologically disturbed by say, a trauma in the family, an argument with a partner or an uncomfortable environment. All these factors will influence the ability to be autonomous and, in this sense, a patient or a client will be disadvantaged. Illness and emotional, psychological and social factors will impair their ability to be autonomous. They may not be able to make clear choices or informed judgements and, therefore, be in the passive position of 'patient in the professional hands of care'. Major principles related to health and social care practice, such as informed consent and paternalism, will be discussed in more detail later but it is worthwhile emphasising the point that the professionals have a privileged position in relation to the people for whom they care. Any profession must uphold the central principle of 'respect for persons' which involves acknowledgement of maximising personal autonomy as far as is possible.

It is reasonable to assume that the same principles of personal autonomy will be central to professional autonomy. Professional groups ought to be self-regulating and, through critical self-appraisal within their profession, be capable of maintaining professional autonomy. Ideally, there ought to be independence of action and judgement without interference from other factors, particularly other professional groups. It is important to remind the reader of Evans' example where the nurse, if adhering rigidly to her professional role and expectations without moral concern for her patients, will be not only other directed by the doctor but limited in professional autonomy. This serves to emphasise the point that autonomy is an ideal and some professions may have a long way yet to go before reaching some level of professional autonomy. Professional groups are influenced by their occupational socialisation process. How the individual perceives his/her professional role will influence to a greater or lesser extent individual moral autonomy, personal values and moral codes. Furthermore, if professional autonomy is ignored, professional control is diminished and personal values and one's own moral autonomy is compromised. Autonomy, whilst ideal, is central to moral integrity and personhood and, therefore, valued. (A person who is not licensed or chartered as a member of a specific profession, will still behave professionally and, therefore, value a level of autonomy).

Being self-determined, having self-respect and formulating a regard for self and others is essential for autonomy. Persons are valued as ends in themselves not as means to achieving those ends. Professional autonomy involves personal moral values shared with the professional moral values. The universalizable moral principle is 'respect for persons'. This, in turn, involves human conduct as reflected through appropriate behaviour both personally and professionally. Without personal responsibility to make decisions as a professional and to act accordingly, autonomy and accountability as professional values are meaningless. The principle of autonomy, from which the idea of informed consent is derived, has only developed recently. Both autonomy and the principle of informed consent will be discussed in much greater detail in Section Two related to research practice.

Health and nursing

Nurses and health care practitioners have a duty to follow the norms, values and goals of their profession. All health care practitioners attempt to preserve public confidence and ought to display a high ethical profile. Adhering to a code of practice helps to enhance this. Often other professionals share this need to preserve public confidence and devise their own specific codes of conduct or practice. Examples can be found within law and applied psychology. Other caring professions, such as social work, are not yet at the stage of explicitly stating their professional ethics and values through a code, although moral values are implicit within their areas of good practice.

Within the nursing and health care field, one professional value that is central is maximising autonomy. This applies to the patients/clients and to the professionals themselves. It involves choosing for oneself, making decisions and in order to exercise autonomy, much will depend upon the amount of information received. It is equally important in education, law, research and psychology. Within nursing, medicine and research, autonomy involves 'informed consent'. Informed consent will be discussed in greater detail in later chapters and in section two. However, it is essential to raise its centrality at the beginning within the health care field of professional ethics. Many others who work with people who may not be members of a specific recognized profession, but in their private and occupational life, behave professionally, will recognize the need for 'professional ethics' in the widest and deepest sense. Midgley (1991b) remarks that moral philosophers , if counting themselves as professional, should be closely concerned with 'real everyday' moral practice, 'practising what we preach'.

Passmore (1984) notes that in only two cases, i.e. medicine and law, the concept of ethics relates to the practice of those professions. Nevertheless changes have occurred within the education and training of the professions generally and we can now claim that nursing and education clearly show established patterns of development in professional ethics.

Education and research

There is no pressure or obligation to become a nurse, doctor, educator or researcher. However, when a professional role is adopted, moral responsibilities automatically become part of being a member of that profession. Inclusion of research is not claiming that a researcher as such is a recognised professional. Nevertheless, if one is a member of a profession, whether in nursing, other health professions, medicine, social care, education, law or management, the professional may, to a greater or lesser degree, be involved in research. Furthermore, research is often viewed as part of the education of professionals, therefore, part of a profession's foundation and growth. The British Psychological Society has devised a code of conduct for practising psychologists and researchers and most nurses will know there is now a code of practice for nursing research. Any researcher in any field that works with people ought to be aware of the ethical implications of research practice. Indeed, some professionals or educationalists spend most of their professional life carrying out research.

According to Passmore, a professional moral code cannot automatically be justified by the fact that a code relates to a special class of persons in virtue of their peculiar relationships to other persons, organisations or activities. Passmore claims that a special moral code is necessary within a profession for one or all of the following reasons:

■ Whilst being a member of a particular profession you may be subjected to temptations. Therefore, it is necessary to protect and warn the professional of such misuse of their professional position

■ Members of a profession may be called in regularly to act in ways which would be beyond the call of duty

■ Members of a profession may be exempt in respect of certain action from moral demands made by others; they may have to ignore considerations which ought normally to be taken into account.

■ An additional reason may also be worth consideration. Professionals have a special access to privileged information and special knowledge acquired through their training and education, as well as through practice. This information and knowledge can, on the one hand, be withheld for a variety of good reasons through practice, i.e. confidentiality or, alternatively, be used inappropriately and unprofessionally (Henry, 1992).

Clearly, nurses and doctors will identify with all the reasons given. Educators particularly and professionals likewise would clearly identify certain areas for a special code of conduct. Generally, in higher education organisations educators wish to achieve and foster communication and advancement of knowledge. Implicit within higher education institutions is the pursuit of moral behaviour through a moral education process. This specifically relates to the vocational role and teaching the profession, itself. The social and moral values may relate to changing the world in pursuit of the greater good. Educators, therefore, have, as Passmore remarked, a reminding code of practice and can relate to some of the above listed reasons. Educators have a moral responsibility to students and fellow professionals to preserve the central principle of 'respect for persons' and, therefore, to maximise autonomy.

Research issues are thematic across professional practice and education. The higher education sector and the professional areas may be seen to be in a privileged position to choose what research to undertake. Most health care and medical professionals are educated within the higher education sector. Therefore, there is a special responsibility to set higher standards of research practice and be fully aware of the social consequences of research. Higher education organisations ought to act as watchdogs for the public interest, especially within the professional fields. Section two deals in more detail with the research issues. Nevertheless, researchers, whatever their professional or educational background, must be made aware of the aspects of professional ethics and appropriate codes of practice or conduct. Researchers have clearly a professional role in considering generally the moral character of what they do. The same may be said for managers of the professions. The next chapter debates particular elements of management and professional ethics and raises issues for further discussion.

References

Blake W (1961). Auguries of Innocence, *Dictionary of Quotations*, p50, Collins, London

Evans M (1991). Professional Ethics and Reflective Practice: A Moral Analysis, Gray E and Pratt R eds, *Towards a Discipline of Nursing*, Churchill Livingstone, London, pp 309–333

Henry C (1992). *Organisational Values in Higher Education*, April Seminar Paper, University of Central Lancashire

Kasey, K (1973).*One flew over the cuckoo's nest*, Pan, London, p255.

Midgley M (1991). Can't we make moral judgement?, Hughes J ed, *Mind Series*, The British Press, London.

Midgley M (1991b). Wisdom, Information and Wonder: What is Knowledge For? Routledge, London and New York.

Milne A A (1926). *Winnie the Pooh*, Metheun, London, p 45

Passmore J (1984). Academic Ethics, *J Applied Philos*, 1, 63–77

Wilcox J (1992). *The Learning Community: A Report on Values and Ethics in Higher Education*, Manhattan College, New York

2 Management and leadership
An ethical debate
Glenys Pashley

*'Thou art weighed in the balance and not found
wanting.........................*   *(Daniel - 5:27)*

*In this chapter, a discussion develops regarding the essential nature
and development of leaders/managers in health care. Whilst the
chapter highlights how important the leader's/manager's role is in
making decisions and supporting appropriate research, it clearly
emphasises the need for them to uphold ethical practice. The chapter
discusses ways in which the managers of the future ought to be educated
or trained in order to raise 'ethical awareness' and improve
managerial practice.*

Never more so than in health care, should management
strategies be researched. Management is about coping with
complexity. Leadership by contrast is about coping with
change and obviously all health care professionals, specifically
nurses, are involve in the latter claim. Setting direction of that
change is fundamental to leadership. The task of leadership
involves values and motivation of people and the allocation of
financial and other resources as set to an overall direction. So
what has this to do with ethics? First, the priority for the health
care areas must be to acquire effective strategic leaders for the
future enhancement of health care. The responsibility of
training and education of these is, therefore, essential.

A leader will be held **accountable** for good ethical practice
but it involves, collectively, professional accountability.
Furthermore, a manager must support the research necessary
to improve practice.

Management and leadership

For Kotter 'management is about coping with complexity...leadership is about coping with change.' This appears to be an arbitrary distinction, since it could be argued that change involves complexity. This may in fact be one reason why Kotter (1990) goes on to suggest that leaders must play a dual role of both manager and leader. Similarly, Zalenzik (1977) contends that managers should exercise leadership qualities because the manager alone tends to preserve the status quo whereas the manager who is also a leader is more likely to change behaviour patterns so that they are more effective. Likewise, Fobbs (1990) argues for a key distinction between leaders and managers. She suggests that leadership involves the influencing of the behaviour of individuals or groups within an organisation and that management is the process through which leadership is accomplished. Perhaps the most striking disparity between management and leadership is summarised in a comment by Bennis (1989), 'the manager does things right, the leader does the right thing.' A more forward looking and positive perspective however is reflected in a statement by Irvin and Michaels (1989) who claim 'doing the right things right' is important to effective leadership. The problem arising from this statement however rests with identifying the right things to do and the right way in which to do them. This issue obviously relates to the task of identifying key competencies involved in effective strategic leadership and the types of leadership training and development which will enhance effective performance. However, it is important to bear in mind Harvey Jones' (1988) implicit but pertinent suggestion that leadership involves both qualities and skills and that management involves only skills. He believes that leadership can be developed to a certain extent but is equally a product of genetics and the socialisation process. This proposition evokes the eternal nature/nurture debate; either we are born with certain qualities or we acquire certain skills through the learning process. As Harvey Jones goes on to comment, many of the characteristics required by leaders can be developed through training but individual limitations will determine the extent to which training can be effective. How then do we develop through training the aspects of the leader of the future. What ethical issues arise, what obligations do we have to manage appropriate change effectively?

Organisational values and applied ethics are central to ways of developing and encouraging an ethical approach to leadership qualities.

Whilst ethics comes down to personal decisions of the leaders and managers, those decisions ultimately affect the organisation, whether it be the hospital or the health care studies college or the community organisation and the leaders therein. A degree of 'trust' in the ethical standards of organisational managers within the health care domain is essential. Organisations must have a commitment to the development of ethical standards. How then does the education of leaders emerge that will influence the ethical perceptions and behaviour of their employees?

Concepts such as empowerment, integrity, honesty, trust, control, authority, power, confidentiality and responsibility, all inherent prescriptive features of the effective strategic leader, have an ethical foundation. Similarly, ethical standards are central to a corporate culture which, in turn, may be influenced by the leader through his/her awareness of organisational behaviour. The leader concerned to initiate, guide and maintain effective and profitable change ought to ensure that decision making does not exclude the ethical concerns. Indeed, in America an ethical corporate culture is seen to enhance strategic advantage. Consequently, there is emphasis now being given to ethics training in order that ethical considerations are integrated into the decision making process throughout the organisation (McDonald and Zepp, 1990). Furthermore, it is the leaders and managers that make the decision in relation to the type of research that is carried out, particularly 'in house' research

A leader/manager should possess values of caring, integrity, self development, trust and co-operation.

These are the ethical issues that may be viewed as essential to the nurse professional/leader/manager now and in the future.

Ethics and the individual leader

Increasing numbers of organisations outside the health field are now devoting time for ethics education and training. If other organisations clearly within a commercial endeavour turn towards ethics, then perhaps the research priority for the National Health Service, with the change towards trust status, is to do likewise. Furthermore, the intent for leaders within the professional field, is to pay direct attention to the universal principle of 'respect for persons' which is clearly central to health care management. From this universal moral principle stems issues of personal integrity, self development common ground and shared values that reflect the leaders and managers of health care practice.

Two major changes to implement levels of ethical practice for the leader within a health care organisation involve:

■ running specific ethics training programmes to enable managers to recognise the ethical component of a management decision

■ employing individuals of adequate and desirable ethical standards

The first point requires a variety of detailed schemes and forms of teaching programmes related specifically to managers and leadership. Concern rests upon the point made in chapter one, that ethics and values are not only of current interest but essential in all aspects of professionalism.

It is often thought that health practitioners and health care managers and leaders are 'doers' and need to achieve effective solutions to practical problems. This may mean that there is little time for reflection or to apply ethical analysis. The role of the applied ethicist or educator who is not necessarily a practitioner is to advise and encourage high levels of understanding and raise the level of awareness for managers and leaders. This involves a partnership between the teacher of ethics and the professional manager/leader. The problem is how we deal confidently with the ethical issues arising in current management and leadership practice in times of great change.

'Ivory tower' principles may have little room in the practical every day management of health care. The universal moral principle of 'respect for persons' must be seen to be reflected through a managers professional behaviour in managing care, and in decision-making and supporting appropriate research. The education and training responsibilities at present require the educational ethicist to teach, train and advise within the organisational setting.

Educational ethicists and the professional managers/ leaders share and trade in values. It is for this reason that the teaching of professional ethics should be introduced into the management's/leaders' curriculum and, second, encourage the partnership between educationalists, researchers and managers in a practical environment. Ethical debates in the classroom situation or through ethics committees may occur periodically. On their own, they are not necessarily effective in the education and decision making process. Therefore, there is a major role for the educational ethicist to act as a practical educator as consultant.

The second point relating to employing ethically-minded leaders is important for the following reasons. The obvious point is to claim that it is easier to employ individuals with appropriate ethical standards and shared organisational values than to try and reshape their standards and skills to become good leaders/managers. Interviewees should be questioned about ethics and organisational values by describing a hypothetical situation and then asking how they would react or respond to it. Reference-checking has always provided verification of information contained in applications forms. Comments on the ethical standards of potential employees could be obtained from the candidate's referees or previous supervisor. Some detail perhaps could be given in relation to appropriate leadership training, as that in itself has ethical implications for success of health care management.

Implications for the training of leaders

It now becomes important to address some of the implications for training and professional development of leaders. Just as there is no single theory of leadership that can provide a blueprint for how an individual should lead, likewise, there is no single training programme that can be specified as being appropriate for all potential or developing leaders. Different types and styles of leadership abound, all of which are influenced by the environment, the work force, the organisation, strategies, desire for change, the role of planning, values, culture, resources, professional background and personalities. Such factors are not static, they are dynamic and, therefore, perhaps the most important quality or skill that a leader can possess or develop is flexibility. It is essential also that leaders find a balance between being task oriented and ensuring the human resources are valued and effectively utilised. As Adair (1983) proposed in his notion of action-centred leadership, effective leadership necessitates being able to create a bond between the task, the individual and the team. To facilitate this bonding appropriately, personal qualities and acquired skills must be evident.

Professional development programmes can be designed to enhance many of the qualities and skills referred to in this discussion and can focus upon:

- challenging broad based assignments to develop the knowledge base and strategic skills — {**Career Maze**}
- lateral jobs moves as well as promotion
- the provision of a mentor who can share knowledge and experience
- group workshops aimed at facilitating communication and interpersonal skills, sensitivity training, peer relations,

assertion skills, confidence building, decision making, problem solving, delegation and team building

■ an understanding of merit rating, i.e. learn to reward the process rather than the results

■ computer based training, video-taped vignettes, case studies

■ improve theoretical knowledge of leadership theory and the array of influential organisational aspects such as culture and values

■ develop an understanding of the relevance of applied psychology, for example, motivations, reward, self concept, perception and individual differences

■ business ethics training

■ role modelling and management by walkabout

■ research practice into NHS management and leadership qualities

An effective strategic leader must constantly review his/her self development through a deliberate process of learning. Leaders are also learners and must recognise that they can learn equally well from mistakes as well as success. Not only should the leader cope with and produce change in the organisation, the processes and the people, but also be committed to changing the self. A starting point for this process of self change may be to identify one's learning style and the associated strengths and weaknesses. Seters and Field (1990) provide a historical review of leadership theory and, through their developmental categorisation, provide a framework consisting of nine ordered eras which can serve to facilitate leaders in identifying at what levels they operate, for example, the cultural era reflects a leader who is influential at the top level and who serves to initiate and change the direction of the organisation. However, Seters and Field conclude by remarking that no single era identified is sufficient to explain the leadership phenomenon, hence the talk of a potential 'integrative era' that links previous knowledge and leads to the development of a conceptual integrating framework which enhances more co-ordinated understanding of what effective leadership means. Perhaps pre-empting the contents of this new integrative era of leadership they propose some qualities and skills that the future practice of leadership will demand:

- visionary
- prepared to take risks
- highly adaptable to change
- delegate authority
- emphasise innovation
- exemplify organisational values, goals and culture
- awareness of influential environmental factors
- new perspective on power
- build the skills and confidence of others
- empower others
- think strategically
- energise others into action
- court a collective view of leadership
- facilitate followers to become leaders and agents of change
- encourage complementary leaders

These last three attributes support the argument for there being more than one leader. Given the vast array of qualities and skills prescribed for the effective strategic leader, it seems inconceivable that leadership can depend upon a single right individual possessing all of these attributes, many of which are mutually exclusive. Further, it is questionable whether a single individual could be developed and trained to possess and employ effectively all of these characteristics. A team of individuals may better meet the criteria for effective strategic leadership. If this were the way forward then teamwork, communication and interpersonal skills would be central and need to focus on pooling experience, information, judgement, qualities and skills. As Kotter (1990) suggests, there is a need for 'lots of leaders all capable of little acts of leadership'. In this constantly changing environment Kotter believes that a single leader is insufficient; competent leaders are required at all levels. To add to this, an underpinning ethical system of practice is required.

Rosener (1990) reports the findings of a survey and remarks that women encourage the building of teams and participation, the sharing of power and information and are more likely than men to make people feel important and energised. Her concept of the androgynous leader may also be relevant; leaders who find a balance between interpersonal sensitivity and task competence. There is a need for a mixture of qualities and skills that both men and women can provide, hence individuals might benefit from joint professional development programmes which focus attention on the positive traits traditionally associated with the opposite sex (Korabik and Ayman, 1989).

Whatever types of training and professional development programmes are introduced, it is important to bear in mind Harvey Jones' contention that such programmes have their limitations. It is debatable whether an individual can learn qualities, but it is accepted that skills can be taught. Given this scenario it would seem sensible to identify some distinction between what competencies are to count as qualities and which are to be regarded as skills. Not only does this have implications for the selection and/or training of individuals for leadership, but also for the content, aims and emphasis of training programmes. In the new age of NHS change, it is crucial that nurse managers/leaders are developed, perhaps substantiated by relevant research into the issues that the new leaders have to face in managing change, (cf Chapter 10).

At this point it is worth making some comments regarding the concept of competencies. It could be argued that competencies arise out of needs and are required to be expressed in terms of clear outcomes which must be met and assessed in the light of standards. A competency based training model could be developed and delivered in a development centre aiming to facilitate leadership potential. It would be essential that potential leaders move across diagonally through a framework or matrix of identified competency needs and also that the acquired skills are transferable. Such a matrix of competencies could be company specific, practical and incorporate the philosophies of 'just in time' and 'total quality management'. Developing competencies might even be perceived as a way of life rather than a short term course of action. However, it is equally important to bear in mind that the concept of competencies has its problems. First, it is questionable whether a competence based development model is a means of ensuring change in individuals. Second, most competencies have different meanings and uses in different social and culture contexts, for example, the competence sensitivity. In this sense the application of national and international training programmes becomes difficult to implement. Third, who assesses the attainment of competencies and who assesses the assessors? Fourth, is the concept of competencies relevant to senior managers and leaders or should there be more emphasis upon a performance profile?

The central problem may not lie with formulating ideal and prescriptive ways in which an individual can set the direction of organisational change, but likely rests with changing the individual into the ideal and effective strategic leader for the purposes of implementing change. There may be a fine line between qualities and skills; the distinction may pose theoretical and semantic problems. On the other hand, the differences may be significant in training and in practice. Further, the terms leader and leadership are labels which are applied to people's behaviour. Labels can be inappropriately attached and are often assumed to have a cause and effect relationship. As Calder (1977) remarks, 'the belief that a certain leadership quality produces a certain behaviour is transformed into the expectation that an instance of the behaviour implies the existence of the quality'. Given that most believe leadership has certain effects the danger lies in simply attributing success or failure to the person and not taking into account the organisation.

Whilst this chapter has discussed in some detail qualities and aspects of leadership styles, it is important to recognise that ethical issues are implicit in all aspects of identifying the leader, educating and training for leadership and organisational values. The health care services and organisations are going through periods of rapid change and what is important is the need for good management and leadership that raises the ethical profile of the organisation. Each organisation can be viewed as a community and within that moral community, awareness of the ethical issues for leadership can help to manage change effectively.

References

Adair J (1983). *Effective Leadership*, Pan, London

Calder B J (1977). An Attribution Theory of Leadership, in Staw B and Salancik G, New Directions in Organisational Behaviour, St Clair Press, Chicago.

Fobbs J (1990) *Enhancing Organisational Vision*, Women in Management Conference, Vienna

Harvey Jones J (1988). *Management and Leadership in Our Society Today and Tomorrow*, The Sir Douglas Glover Memorial Lecture

Korabik K and Ayman R (1989). Should women managers have to act like men? *J Manag Dev*, 8, 6, 23–32.

Kotter J P (1990). What leaders really do, *Harvard Bus Rev*, May–June 1990, pp103–111.

McDonald G M and Zepp R A (1990). What should be done? A practical approach to business ethics, *Manag Decision*, 28, 1, 9–14.

Rosener J B (1990). Ways women lead, *Harvard Bus Rev*, Nov–Dec 1990, pp119–125.

Seters D A and Field R H G (1990). The evolution of leadership theory, *J Contemp Manag*, 3, 3, 29–45.

Change management process
Ethical approaches in a macro perspective

Laurie Wood

The art of progress is to preserve order amid change and to preserve change amid order.... (Alfred North Whitehead).

Whilst chapter two highlights important ethical issues that may enhance good leadership practice within NHS organisations, this chapter identifies ethical issues from a macro perspective. Part of the sensible 'thing to do' in managing change is to look towards providing 'good education' for those who manage change, and, in turn, those who make decisions regarding supporting or preventing 'in house' research. Nevertheless, prior to health care research, some understanding is needed of how the macro structure and process of organisational change comes into being. Research on how and what influences the organisational structure is often necessary for this sort of understanding. This chapter and the previous chapter lay down the foundations and gives some 'food for thought' on the 'nature of the beast'.

This chapter clearly identifies some ethical issues and enhances the 'need' for research in the field of Health Care Management. Health care managers, regardless of origin, either from clinical professional practice or other fields, are members of the organisation's community and are more accountable than ever before on how they 'manage' the delivery of care.

Introduction

In managing change within public sector organisations, ethical issues are of paramount importance. Nowhere has this been more clearly demonstrated than in the most recent radical changes to the NHS. Theories of change management focus largely on the organisation and the role of its internal structure and processes in gaining commitment to change. However, research has shown that this cannot be achieved successfully in isolation, without first considering the role of the organisation within the broader 'macro' environment.

This chapter examines the approach to NHS reforms from the macro perspective, against a background of accepted management theories in order to draw lessons for ethical approaches to future public sector reforms.

Background to NHS Reforms

Since the end of the second World War, and particularly in the last decade, the pace of social change has accelerated sharply. For the NHS, external environment changes have been, and continue to be, significant, in the form of changing population patterns, the growing salience of health care as a public policy issue, technological and medical advancements, and externally imposed constraints on expenditure. Typical of most public sector organisations, the basic bureaucratic structure of the NHS caused its response to such environmental changes to be prolonged. This situation could not be sustained. The NHS needed to adjust more readily if it was to survive politically, as a universal, free at the point of delivery healthcare system, into the 1990s. This also emphasises the important value, a western society places upon a welfare system.

The nature of change

The government aimed to create a new market-led management culture within the NHS in order to control public spending and become more responsive to health service needs. In accordance with coincident trends in our society, this was to be achieved through a strategic policy of centralising control over decision-making whilst decentralising activity. This would continue the move from hierarchic top-down organisations to looser constellations and networks.

It also chose to adopt a revolutionary[1], rather than evolutionary, approach to implementation[2.] The experiences of key parties in this process provide useful lessons for managing radical change successfully within the public sector. The question arises, is it an ethical system of managing change; are individuals viewed through 'economic eyes' as cost units instead of persons?

The nature of the organisation

A study of organisational theory makes it apparent that for the government to implement its planned changes within the NHS, the process would be inevitably be constrained by the organisational structure itself. The Health Service is 'a **rationally structured system** of interrelated activities' (Clifton-Williams 1978), and can also be classified in Weber's terms (1947) as a **bureaucracy** i.e. a rational organisation, with clear and formal regulations and responsibilities, and authority clearly, explicitly and formally divided and distributed.

According to Weber[3] (1947), in these circumstances it is likely that behaviour would be based on analysis, calculation and procedures, and, as such, would be predictable but can we do this within a community of professionals? In practice, within the NHS, many conflicts exist which serve as barriers to the rational process; political priorities, balancing opposing interests eg. those of clinicians and managers, power politics and hidden agenda. This pattern is typical of many public sector organisations.

The McKinsey 7S framework provides a useful model for highlighting the need for *internal* consistency between strategy, structure, systems, skills, staff, management strategy

[1]This approach requires certain management principles to be observed in order to achieve a successful reform, discussed later in this chapter.

[2]Whether this radicalism was a consequence of the Thatcherite ideology, or the underlying social changes that made Thatcherism possible has been a subject of debate (Marxism Today, October, 1988).

[3]Weber makes a distinction between 'formal' rationality, which relates to methodology and 'substantive' rationality which relates to outcomes; how we make assessments and calculate outcomes and how they work in reality.

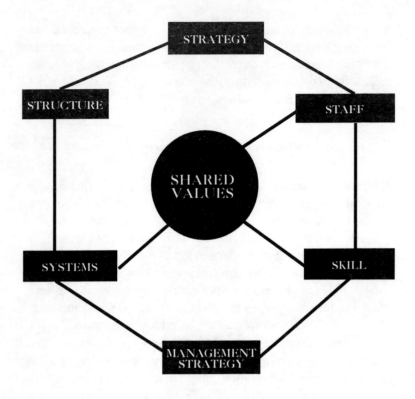

Fig. 3.1 McKinsey 7S framework

and shared values. Many organisations attempt to follow this
model in successfully implementing change; However. it has
been suggested by Mintzberg (1983) that 'true' fit, between an
organisation and its environment, can only be achieved
through **internal** and **external** consistency.

It is helpful, then, to view the NHS organisation as a system
of a collection of interrelated elements where a change in one
element will lead to ramifications elsewhere. If these elements
are to work together towards a shared goal, a joint and flexible

[4]The 1983 Griffiths Report and subsequent White Papers could be seen as
a catalyst to achieving internal consistency. The general management
structure recommended by the Griffiths Report, with its emphasis on
leadership and communication, was aimed at consistency, but ultimately
suffered from an illogical cultural fit or lack of shared values.

response to environmental changes is required. Also, the 'openness' and multi-layed structure of this system should not

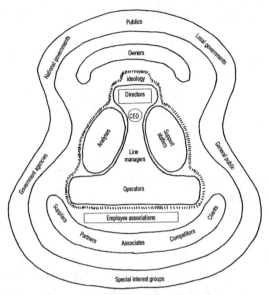

Fig. 3.2 Mintzberg's organisational system

be ignored if effective change management is to be successfully implemented.[4]

The characteristics of Not-for-Profits (NFP's)

Building on this work, Mintzberg (1983) produced evidence to suggest the presence of particular internal power structures in Not-For-Profit organisations. These were missionary and meritocracy. Of these, the **meritocracy** most closely relates to the existing structure of the NHS.

Table 3.1. Mintzberg's 'meritocracy'

Main characteristics
hospitals, universities and other professional bureaucracies
power resides with the experts in the operating core: experts owe allegiance to their profession, rather than the particular organisation
complex mission leads to weak CEO power and displacement of organisational goals by the goals of the experts (autonomy, excellence)

Source: Bowman C and Asch D (1987). *Strategic Management*, Macmillan, London

The significant strategic ramifications of this type of organisational structure are:

■ NFP often dependent on scarce, highly-mobile professionals

■ NFP can be indirectly controlled externally by the professional's associations. Does this give too much power to the professional bodies or does it ensure ethical practice, in that those who control are held accountable to professional codes of practice?

■ political behaviour encouraged by goal ambiguity and performance measurement problems: budgets allocated in part on the basis of the perceived power of departments

■ professional bodies can act through their members to impede the introduction of strategic changes (rigidity in defence of professional norms)

■ strategic change **usually** comes about through persuasion and negotiation.

These factors, identified by Mintzberg, are important in helping to evaluate the ethical methods adopted by the government of implementing strategic change within the NHS, since the management of change may be significantly enhanced or hindered by the management of those external factors which influence key interest key groups- ie. the 'stakeholders'.

Change strategies in public services

In theoretical terms, the emphasis required by government represented a radical shift in internal power structures towards a private sector model, with accountability for public sector finance replacing the 'commercial' objective. However, the structural analysis has shown that no matter how commercially oriented the *board* of the NHS might become, as a public service it would still be a fundamentally different form of organisation from the private sector firm. A major ethical issue is apparent in imposing private sector forces upon public sector organisations.

The importance of stakeholders and coalitions

The concept of a coalition of stakeholders (Cyert and March, 1963) is important if an appropriate ethical model is to be developed for the communication of change programmes within public sector organisations. Freeman (1984) argues that to survive in the future, organisations must deal actively with their stakeholders. The 'stakeholder' concept encompasses all those people who have an interest in the enterprise and may seek to influence its future - customers, consumers, pressure groups, investors, the media, suppliers, competition, the trade, the community, legislators etc.. Interest groups of external stakeholders or 'publics' are specific to each organisation. They must be determined as the initial step in understanding the interaction process.

Defining external stakeholders

Few examples of stakeholder analysis exist for the purposes of understanding influences on organisational change within public service organisations. Pratt and Lockwood (1985) provide an interesting model of the external stakeholders affecting the University sector of Higher Education, which is a helpful illustration of the various forces acting upon a public sector organisation. It has been adapted here to reflect the interest groups and pressures acting upon the NHS.

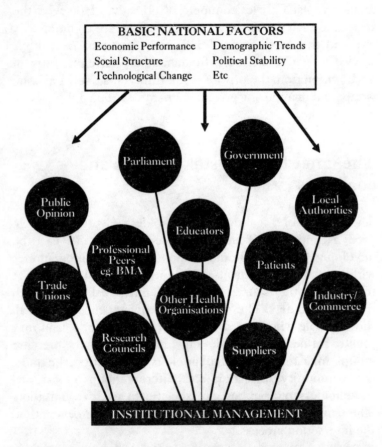

Source: Adapted from Lockwood and Davies (1985), P4

Fig 3.4 External bodies influencing the NHS

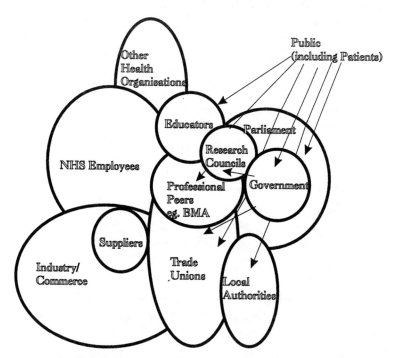

Figure 3.5: Key Stakeholder Domains (External Stakeholder Groups in the Management of NHS Change

However, these spheres of influence are not mutually exclusive, as Pratt and Lockwood imply. For example, within the NHS, a BMA doctor may also be an NHS 'customer', a union member, even a political activist. He may also be a member of several networks - associates, of family, of social friends, as well as a member of the general public. If the stakeholder concept is to be relevant to the changemakers from a communications perspective, then the nature of these relationships must be investigated further to understand the underlaying interactions.

Firstly, to identify the key domains, the groups must be viewed in terms of their mutual membership- and influence;

[5]A detailed empirical study of the effectiveness of government communications prior to the reform implementation has been undertaken by the author.

In the NHS example, the spheres *central* to the stakeholder network are represented by the professional groups eg. BMA and trade unions. These influence government through parliament, and also employees, industry and the public as opinion leaders in their professional status, via the media.

For public sector organisations, the influence of these bodies on the attitude and opinion of the general public is of particular importance for the following reasons:

■   the model demonstrates that public opinion will have a direct influence on employees and other key groups.

■   the public are not only 'customers' but also, inter alia, the service owners.

■   their collective influence may affect both the acceptance and continuity of change, even ultimately via the democratic process.

In radical change management of public services, the body which can harness *popular* support will ultimately succeed in its objectives. Furthermore, their values will be essential in influencing delivery of service.

Government management of key stakeholders in the NHS

Returning to the NHS situation, the government's management of key stakeholders groups is now reviewed, based on the events of the time[5]. A campaign of opposition to the Bill began in earnest with the publication of the White Paper. The plans had been leaked to the media in advance by Mr. Robin Cook, Shadow Health Spokesman, and were subjected to a continuous barrage of opposition from representatives of the British Medical Association, the medical Royal Colleges and other health groups. An NHS Support group was established to coordinate the activities of opposing groups, in particular the BMA representing 32,000 General Practitioners, the Royal Colleges, consultants and leaders of the 25 organisations which together represent the 500,000

NHS staff. By July 1990, the BMA alone had reputedly spent the best part of £3m opposing the reforms in a carefully planned manner (FT, 28th June 1990 and 11th July 1990). Criticisms were fierce and very public. In an interview on BBC Radio 4, in March 1990, Kenneth Clarke commented:

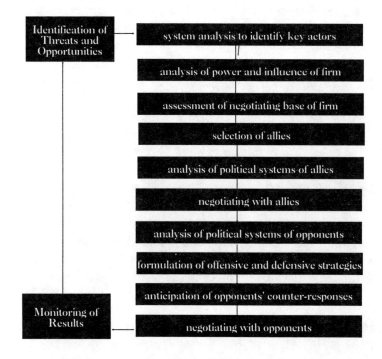

Fig. 3.6 Schematic outline of political strategy formulation

There has been far too much campaigning against these reforms, raising ridiculous fears.

These fears were apparently confirmed with the announcement of up to 1000 job losses by two of the first wave of self-governing hospital trusts, within a month of their change of status in April 1991. (FT. 9th May 1991). Coming on the heels of charging for eyesight tests and dental check-ups, the government's case had not been helped by the vagueness of the White Paper, which left scope for misinterpretation and propaganda, and the coincident unpopularity of the poll tax. Consequently, the government experienced a humiliating defeat in the Monmouth by-election in May 1991. (FT. 15th May 1991)

The case was also not helped by the suggestion that NHS providers, themselves, has a vested interest in highlighting their weaknesses, since these arguments are often used internally to make the case for extra resources. As Enoch Powell, a former Health Minister once wrote:

> *One of the most striking features of the NHS is the continual, deafening chorus of complaint which rises day and night from every part of it, a chorus only interrupted when someone suggests that a different system altogether might be preferable .... it presents what must be a unique spectacle of an undertaking that is run down by everyone engaged in it (Economist, 21st May, 1988).*

Against this background of mounting adverse public opinion and consequent stakeholder influence, research suggests that any internal management of change initiative would almost inevitably face staunch opposition. The identification of what is given priority in relation to values held by political parties, influence structure and process.

Political strategies in the public sector

From the NHS experience, it is apparent that due to the influence of stakeholder and coalitions, concentration on internal change management and the application of theories developed for the private sector is not sufficient to develop a positive dynamic for change in the Public Sector.

Slatter (1984), for example, identifies eight key actions needed to implement a recovery strategy, in which the **establishment of communications** with key stakeholders in order to gain credibility is given high priority.

[6]Plant R (1987) identified the italicised items as key elements of the change process in *Managing Change and Making it Stick*, Fontana Collins, London.

This theme has been developed more recently by Macmillan and Jones (1986), who provide a model for political strategy formulation. The stages are particularly appropriate, and could have usefully been applied in this case.

Ineffective political strategies may explain why it has been historically difficult to introduce into the public sector. March and Olsen (1989) provide an insight:

> *The state affects society as well as being affected by it, and can itself be seen as a structured institutionalised order, with its own standard operating procedures, values and distribution of power.*

Conclusion

Theory suggests that communications strategies must be applied to 'stakeholders' groups. Strategies should target not only internal stakeholders, but more importantly, in the context of radical organisational change within the public sector, should extend beyond the organisation to the external change agents. It should be a matter of priority and ethical responsibility for such organisations to positively involve the external stakeholders at an early stage to protect the continuity of change, with evidence of the need for **concern** for the public, **integrity** and dialogue to create **credibility** before **visibility**. This is essential for good ethical practice in managing change.

It is postulated that in the case of the NHS, government having *recognised the need* for change, failed *to mobilise commitment of the 'critical mass'* for the changes it proposed; almost inevitably given the 'culture shock' approach to implementation. It failed **to build a shared vision**, in particular to harness stakeholder opinion, thereby putting the continuity of the change at risk. It chose to ignore *the current reality* and thereby constrained its ability to *'get there'*[6].

Hence, in public sector organisations, the issues of managerial effectiveness and democratic involvement must extend **beyond** the organisation, for only with the commitment and support of the external stakeholders and their ethical/moral values and identified priorities for reform, can management feel secure in implementing any change as a long-term strategy, as opposed to a politically-motivated short-term tactic.

References

Alford R (1975). *Health Care Politics.* University of Chicago Press, London

Alleway L (1987). Back on the Outside Looking In. *Health Serv J,* 16th July, 818-819.

Bowman C and Asch D (1987). *Strategic Management.* Macmillan, London

Butler R J and Wilson D C (1989). *Managing Voluntary and Non-profit Organisation: Strategy and Structure.* Routledge, London

CM 555 (1989) *Working for Patients.* HMSO, London

Cyert R M and March J G (1963). *A Behavioural Theory of the Firm.* Prentice Hall, New Jersey

Economist (1988). Health Service: Opting Out, *Economist.* 21st May, 41

Financial Times (1990). The Politics of NHS Reform. *Financial Times.* 18th June, 18

Financial Times (1990). Doctors Plan Offensive against Health Reforms. *Financial Times* 28th June, 8

Financial Times (1990). A New Era for the NHS. *Financial Times* 3rd July, 8

Financial Times (1990). Clarke Hints at Alternative Medicine, *Financial Times* 11th July, 9

Kerr H (1991). The Problem of Presentation that dogs the Tory Party, *Financial Times* 9th May, 12.

Forster D and Hadley R (1989). Conditions of Successful Change. *Health Ser Manag,* October, 215-218.

Lockwood G (1985). Universities as Organisations. Lockwood G and Davies J eds, *Universities: The Management Challenge.* NFER Nelson Windsor

Macmillan I C and Jones P (1986). *Strategy Formulation: Power and Politics* (2nd ed), West Publishing Company, St Paul, Minnesota

Mintzberg H (1983). *Power In and Around Organisations*. Prentice Hall New Jersey.

Newman W H and Wallender H W (1983). Managing Not- For- Profit Enterprises, Parson RJ ed, *The Management Process: A Selection of Readings for Librarians*. American Library Association, Chicago.

Pratt J and Lockwood G (1985). The External Environment in Lockwood G and Davies J eds, *Universities: The Management Challenge*, NFER Nelson, Windsor.

Slatter S 1984, *Corporate Recovery*, Penguin Harmondsworth.

Times (1989). Anger at Cook Leak of NHS Reform Plans, *Times*, 28th Jan, 1

Weber M (1947). *The Theory of Social Economic Organisation*. Free Press, Glencoe.

Related forms of knowledge
An ethical approach
Christine Henry and Glenys Pashley

Does it matter? — losing your legs
For people will always be kind..(Siegfried Sassoon 1886–1967)

Chapters two and three deal with some major issues that arise from management perspectives at both micro and macro level. These very important integrated areas of concern must be considered prior to 'health care research' being undertaken within the NHS community. The previous chapters give a generalised profile necessary for prior understanding, whereas this chapter introduces some of the ethical issues that arise from application of a 'knowledge base' that professionals within the NHS have. Whilst this chapter again gives a different, but nevertheless, generalised profile of ethical issues, it emphasises the complexity, and yet the importance of an ethical theme or system, integrated within health care delivery and professional practice. There are some issues raised concerning the professionals' curriculum and aspects of biological sciences, social and behavioural sciences are discussed. The chapter clearly emphasises the importance of an integrated ethical curriculum for health care practitioners.

Knowledge essential for health care

A balance has been sought between the biological sciences and the social sciences within the curriculum, particularly for the health care professionals. Generally, the areas of knowledge that the caring professions have studied and applied have broadened conceptions of professional care. Henry and Tuxill (1987) remark that running parallel to this more diverse use of forms of knowledge is 'the view that the individual person is the central character for concern' (p 245).

In other words, central to health and social care practice is 'respect for persons'. This can be identified in areas such as education with student centred learning, in social work, client centred care and in nursing, the nursing process and primary care. This emphasises aspects of personal autonomy as a major ethical concern which in turn focuses upon personhood and respect for persons..

The biological sciences

It is necessary to discuss briefly the biological sciences in relation to health care because of the important aspect for competent professional practice. The biological sciences are, in part, foundational for doctors, nurses and other health professions. A firm understanding of the human biological sciences can and will formulate part of the framework for enhancing the efficient practitioner. However, it is important to remember that for nurses in particular it ought not to be viewed as the central body of knowledge foundational for practice.

Henry and Tuxill remark that there is an uneasy relationship within the curriculum between the biological and social sciences and this reflects the questions surrounding what constitutes science and the forms of knowledge that might accrue more status in areas of certainty and truth. There is the more obvious problem when application of such biological knowledge through practice views the individual person entirely as an organic organism. The aspect of 'choosing' only applies to human beings, i.e. persons and it involves autonomy. It sounds absurd to speak of bacterium or a biological organism exercising choice. Choice is one of many attributes humans like to reserve for themselves (Gregory, 1987, p 147). The problem that arises when viewing the person as just a biological organism can raise important ethical concerns. It does not allow aspects of autonomy to be considered. The patient clearly is viewed as passive.

Furthermore, it raises issues of informed consent. Informed consent will be discussed in greater detail in chapter six. However, it is important to remember that if the patient is viewed as passive what constitutes informed consent is left to the health practitioner to decide and he or she will have special access to professional areas of knowledge that may not be given to patients. Patients may be viewed as passive and, therefore, not capable of understanding.

What the profession values will determine what it does and, if the biological sciences are valued as the central body of knowledge, then it will influence in turn the professional practice. Different professions have different roles, norms and goals. Furthermore, the curriculum is central to the education of the professional. The curriculum will, therefore, influence the construction of values the professional will have. Knowledge in itself and understanding of that knowledge is a value for the profession in order to influence good practice. Medicine is centrally focused upon the natural sciences. The biological and physiological sciences are given priority. However, even in medicine, other values, both personal and professional, must ensure some balance through practice and application.

Underpinning the biological sciences is a reductionist and causal model that fits well with aspects of experimental research. However, the positivist model of science does not leave room for non-descriptive value terms such as 'personhood'. The term person is not a technical or a scientific descriptive term and, therefore, cannot be placed appropriately within the natural science domain, nor would we want to place the term as a neutral objective term, relating to a 'fact'. It is value laden. However, the nurse or the medical practitioner relates to the person in their care and the appropriate way in which she or he applies her/his knowledge base as a tool or a process to improve the well being of the person is important to professional practice. Understanding and application of only one form of knowledge, even if valued as central, is not sufficient. The curriculum must also address other forms of knowledge to enhance professional practice.

The term person in common sense terms is used interchangeably with the term 'human'. Moreover, a common sense viewpoint, alone, is not sufficient for the caring professions' curriculum, particularly in respect of actions taken and decisions made through practice. There is a need for sound curriculum development in other disciplines, i.e. social sciences, psychology and ethics. The major concern is that any profession that uses a biological frame of reference, particularly centred on practice of the profession must review the ethical issues and concerns of personhood. In this sense, the term person is a moral concept like the term 'good'. Ethics becomes a major aspect for the analysis values and, therefore, should be part of the curriculum.

Passmore (1978) remarks that science can help us understand individuals even though it does not mention them. This is precisely why levels of awareness must be raised regarding the ethical implications for practice and looking for a balance within the curriculum for professionals. Passmore states:

> *A psychotic classification system does not of itself tell us that Jones is a manic-depressive but it does tell what we have to find out about Jones in order to determine whether he is a manic depressive (Passmore, 1978, p 71).*

The example given by Passmore can apply to the medical classification system or model within the physical illness domain. The example serves to emphasise that underpinning psychiatric and psychological disorders there is a medical model that dominates. According to Passmore, it does not enable us to anticipate in detail the character of Jones' fantasies or determine the etiology of his disorder but it can still help us to understand Jones and perhaps cure him. However, is does not allow us to understand Jones as a person and value him as such and this is why science as a form of knowledge alone is not sufficient for the practitioner of any discipline.

Passmore remarks that science does not replace the concrete; it helps us to understand it (Passmore, 1978, p 72). Likewise, emphasising that the professionals' curriculum should have other forms of knowledge such as social sciences, psychology and ethics involves not only raising levels of awareness but helps us to understand our own values and interpersonal behaviour within the social and professional fields.

Each form of enquiry will offer its own kind of understanding. If we say that a person is X we cannot presume that's all we can say. Science as a form of enquiry will think in general terms. This is perfectly acceptable when applied within the appropriate context. However, if we think of persons as entities in general terms it is morally unacceptable and not in any way sensible within the professional fields of care. There is the example of applying economic science as the only perspective in aspects of health service management where people are counted as costs units (cf Chapter 3).

Henry and Tuxill point out that biologists and natural scientists should take a philosophical look at their subject. This would encourage more awareness. Doctors as a profession ought to encourage ethics within the curriculum. Perhaps more useful to the profession would be postgraduate educational courses. Although doctors may state that 'cure' is central to practice, likewise 'caring' is central to the profession. Nurses and other health professionals ought to highlight the centrality of ethical awareness and issues implicit within their knowledge base in practice. The nurse practitioner may use and apply the biological sciences but they are clearly the patient's/client's advocate. Looking at the concept of personhood and respect for persons is and ought to be an integrated part of the health professional's curriculum. Furthermore, it ought to be a way of strengthening links between the biological and social behavioural sciences.

Social behavioural sciences and ethics

Henry and Tuxill remark that the social sciences viewed from one particular perspective is more predisposed to use the terms 'person' in a unified and meaningful way. This is partly because the term person has, clearly, a social element in relation to its construction and status within society. Furthermore, persons have social features and moral values are involved, such as rights and respect. One only needs to be reminded of Germany's treatment of groups of people during World War Two. Viewed from one particular sociological perspective, a whole ethnic group of people where stripped of their 'personhood' by denying them social identity, rights, freedom of choice, welfare and social interaction. Present day sociological studies advocate that individuals are not social units in a structural sense but emphasise the dangers of denying individuals 'person features' within institutions such as hospitals, schools and prisons. Social sciences have taken on a more interpretative approach.

Roles, norms, and authority

However, there is danger in holding rigidly to professional roles and organisational norms. In the book and the film *One Flew Over the Cuckoo's Nest*, not only did the nurse, institutionalised by her role, exercise rigidly the power that her professional role gave her, but also became the authority on who should and who should not have 'rights' of freedom of choice and respect. Her patients were controlled, portrayed as being often passive and lacking in personal autonomy.

A further example relating to the concept of authority within the hospital setting is given through the experimental study carried out in nurse physician relationships by Hofling *et al* (Mechanic, 1980). The researchers constructed an incident regarding an irregular order from a doctor to a nurse for her to administer a dose of medication. (For reasons of safety a placebo was used.) The nurse was asked to give an excessive dose of medicine. The medication was ordered over the telephone which violated hospital policy and the drug was not authorised or cleared for use. The nurse was not familiar with the doctor's voice. The results showed that 21 of the total 22 subjects would have given the medication. This not only shows the 'power of authority' accepted by one profession over another, but clearly raises ethical issues relating to carrying out such studies by non members of a profession on uninformed members of an identified profession. Furthermore, it emphasises clearly that all professionals need to address ethical practices and raise levels of awareness relating to practice inter-professionally and within research practice.

Psychology

Henry and Tuxill point out that some theories in psychology are within the positivist tradition, e.g. neurosciences and behaviourism. The behaviourist approach may be useful and relevant in understanding processes of learning but the concern lies with persons and respect for persons not rats or cats in puzzle boxes.

There are other perspectives within psychology that may be more relevant for the curriculum. Social, cognitive, humanist, psychodynamic and phenomenological approaches are just some of the approaches that attempt at understanding the person within the health care setting, this includes the area of applied psychology referred to as health psychology. Health psychology will utilise various psychological approaches useful specifically for health care.

With some qualification, it may be suggested that the social sciences have developed into two broad and disparate areas of study, namely the positivist and the humanist approaches. In psychology, generally in line with the positivist tradition, are approaches such as neuroscience, psychobiology, behaviourism, psychometrics and experimental psychology which includes artificial intelligence. Within these approaches there is little room for a unified concept of the person.

It is debatable as to whether neurosciences and psychobiology are clearly within a psychological framework. Both approaches have similar forms of enquiring and conceptual models akin to the biological sciences. Gabriel (1980) remarks that it was Watson, a notable behaviourist who changed psychology from the study of consciousness to the study of behaviour. It was not until the early 1950s with the developments of the more humanistic, cognitive and phenomenological approaches that psychology was viewed as more than the study of behaviour developing full circle and returning, in part, to the study of consciousness (Henry, 1986).

Much like neurosciences and psychobiology, behaviourism was seen to be an objective science. However, there are problems that can arise within the curriculum if the main focus is upon only one psychological approach. For example, extreme behaviourism sees the individual purely as a stimulus response model and the intervening organism, i.e. the individual, is ignored because internal representations cannot be observed. The person is viewed as a reactor to stimuli. Once again, the person is not interactive only a passive reactor to stimuli. There is a danger of taking it as an extremely useful form of psychological management which fits nicely with a medical model in that the person is an object to manipulate. Within the psychobiological and neuroscience areas there is little room for conceptualising personhood. In part, the approaches may allow understanding without mentioning the individual but they ought to be only one part of a part of a body of knowledge useful for the professional's curriculum. There has been a different emphasis placed upon applied psychology recently in order to encompass a more diverse viewpoint and avoid the mechanistic and dehumanising views that materialise with focusing only upon the positivist approach.

The humanist movement, as opposed to the positivist tradition, sees the individual as more active, responsible and free. An extreme humanistic approach has been claimed to be more of an ethical science where person concepts are value laden, not easily defined and cannot be measured or quantified, e.g. concept of 'empathy'. The humanist approach deals with human features such as intentionality, meanings and interpretation.

Idiosyncratic constructs and some social cognitive models deal with experience and ways of thinking. Exploring the psychological models is not the purpose of this chapter, but perhaps it should be restated that although the humanist approach has problems relating to definition of loose concepts, it can be grounded in a phenomenological framework which is more consistent with a psychology of the person (Henry, 1986).

Similarly, in sociology some particular approaches lend themselves to be more relevant for the concept of personhood, e.g. the interactionist approach and ethnomethodology. Some areas of sociology overlap with social psychology particularly when studying various aspects of role, attitude and social perception.

Balance within the curriculum is important and the emphasis upon social sciences on either a psychology or sociology of the person is not disregarding other approaches in the positivist tradition. They are still useful conceptual schemes for understanding particular aspects of the individual.

Nursing knowledge

Nursing knowledge is still in its infancy, Anderson (1991) remarks that theory is derived from practice is still debated at great length and still with some confusion. The traditional view within western culture relating to research and creating a body of knowledge denies the validity of methods and products of thinking that arises from action taken through practice. However, from a professional point of view, it is very difficult to divorce thinking, knowing and action.

One of the ways to influence professional acknowledgement for nursing is through having a specific body of knowledge. Nursing research must generate a specific body of knowledge. Nursing is claimed to be both an art and a science (West, 1991). To qualify this, it is perhaps sensible to say nursing is an applied science in the broadest sense of the term, and because of the central role of 'care' and 'respect for persons' is an 'ethical science' .

Neyle and West (1991) state that there are three distinct areas of science involved and these are:

■   traditional science which includes physics, chemistry, anatomy, physiology and microbiology. The traditional sciences are within the same conceptual frameworks as the biological sciences. Neyle and West state that health professionals borrow from these areas

■   the behavioural and social sciences such as sociology and psychology education and communication studies. According to Neyle and West, these areas of knowledge contribute to the practice of nursing

■   nursing as a science itself. This is viewed as unique to the discipline and results from nursing practice. This is the pursuit of professional practice and professional recognition. The author would also add to the three defined areas of knowledge and identify that ethical domains relate across the three areas and formulate a unified theme crucial to professional practice. Applied nomative or practical ethics ought to be part of the three areas within the curriculum

Traditional sciences have their own rules and methods of enquiry. They involve scientific methodology relating to research practice. However, whilst the scientific form of enquiry is useful as a form of enquiry it ought not to be rigidly viewed as the only form if enquiry central to nursing practice and research.

It may be tentatively claimed that knowing the scientific basis of the possible cause can bring pre-conceived ideas about care.

In respect of professional practice and in the delivery of care, transferable knowledge, that can be applied through practice, is important. A balance is required with greater emphasis given to the effects rather than just the causes of disease.

The nursing curriculum has, by tradition, tended to use the scientific basis of medicine. The modern curriculum reflects a balance by introducing the behavioural, social and ethical sciences. However, emphasis given to one area of knowledge and that area of knowledge remaining central, constrains and damages the pursuit of knowledge.

To conclude Nozick (1981) states, 'values enter into the very definition of what a fact is, the realm of facts cannot be defined or specified without utilising certain values' (p 535).

If this is the case, then there is not such a dichotomy between different forms of knowledge. Scientific objective forms of enquiry, perhaps dealing with facts and the more loosely value laden social sciences could be closely aligned with the underlying themes of values and, in turn, the ethical concerns for professional practice.

References

Anderson B (1991). Mapping the terrain of the discipline, Gray G and Pratt R eds, *Towards a Discipline of Nursing*, Churchill Livingstone, London, pp 95–125

Gabriel C (1980). The development of psychology as a science, Radford J and Govier E eds, *A Textbook of Psychology*, Sheldon Press, London

Gregory R (1987). *Mind in Science: A History of Explanations in Psychology and Physics*, Penguin, London

Henry I C (1986) Conceptions of the Nature of Persons, *Unpublished PhD thesis*, Leeds University

Henry I C and Tuxill C (1987). Concepts of the person: Introduction to the health professional's curriculum, *J Adv Nurs*, **12**, 2245–249

Mechanic D (1980). *Readings in Medical Sociology*, Free Press, London, pp 434–445

Neyle D and West S (1991). In support of a scientific basis, Gray G and Pratt R eds, *Towards a Discipline of Nursing*, Churchill Livingstone, London, pp 265–284

Nozick R (1981). *Philosophical Explanations*, Clarendon Paperbacks, Oxford

Passmore J (1978). *Science and its Critics*, Duckworth, London

Ethical issues

5

in nursing research

Julie Apps and Mags Yeomans

'....three basic principles conferring autonomy, beneficence and justice. But to whom, exactly do these principles apply, and on what basis?......p353, E R Winkler.

Chapter four deals with some of the issues that arise if the curriculum for all health care practitioners, including the medics, is not balanced. Furthermore, it discusses and highlights the need for an ethical theme binding together forms of knowledge within the curriculum, in order to ennhance 'good practice'. However, this chapter specifically addresses issues that arise through carrying out nursing research. It begins by stating that health care research is central in expanding boundaries of knowledge and understanding. It raises issues that must be addressed from a moral standpoint, in relation to research practice by nurses themselves.

Health care research is central to the quest for an increased understanding, improved knowledge and generalised explanation of the complexities of all health related issues. These concepts are fundamental to the education of carers in order to influence and enhance the care delivered to clients both in the clinical setting and in the community. Implicit within this arena is the necessity for those responsible for education to acquire the skills to carry out research and facilitate these skills in others.

Research and ethical considerations are inextricably linked. The researcher must consider the implications of the proposed research, primarily for the participating subjects, but also the resulting status of knowledge and its relevance to society as a whole. Schrock (1984), for example, states that not all research activities lead to an increase in knowledge. In relation to the participants, Burnard and Morrison (1990) remind us that we have no intrinsic right to undertake research.

They go on to say that fundamental issues should be explored at all stages of the research process. These could include the right of the researcher to ask questions and expect responses; the relevance of these questions; are they important or appropriate? As Duffy (1985) also comments, there is an overemphasis in health care research on the quantitative approach, this method often being inadequate in answering important health-related questions. No matter what is done, if an answer to a question such as, 'what is nursing?' is required, empirical research, which takes its principles from the scientific domain, can make only a limited contribution. Duffy (1985) argues that a quantitative approach, which relies on the 'true experiment', is positivistic and she acknowledges the need to include qualitative methodology which takes into account the environmental and social factors affecting the person.

Nursing and midwifery research deals with people in diverse situations, where respect for persons within research **must** be central. This respect can easily be betrayed with the possibility of physical, psychological or social exploitation of the subjects whilst in the pursuit of knowledge and the fact that much of the success of research depends on prying into other people's activities (Schrock, 1984). The researcher must take this into account in the planning stage. Schrock (1984) also points out that nursing research is a costly and time consuming activity, which leads us to the financial aspect of research, in itself worthy of ethical consideration. Downie and Calman (1989) say that, for the researcher, the source of money may lead to moral dilemmas. An example of this would be the researcher comparing the patient's ability to work on different forms of renal treatment, the research sponsored by a firm who make peritoneal dialysis fluid. Would the researcher examine the benefits of this treatment in a more favourable light to secure continued funding and perhaps employment?

Having reviewed some of the general issues in planning research, it is important to consider how the researcher can work towards maintaining his/her own professional integrity and also protect the intrinsic rights of the research respondents.

Nursing research, compared with other disciplines, is in its infancy — the earliest guidelines on ethical values being published by the American Nurses' Association (ANA) in 1968. Similar guidelines were produced by the Canadian Nurses' Association (CNA) in 1972, with the Royal College of Nursing (RCN) following with a more comprehensive approach in 1977. In 1985, the International Council of Nurses issued *Guidelines for Nursing Research Development*, which recognised the rights of the individual. On its inception in 1984, the United Kingdom Central Council for Nursing, Midwifery and Health Visiting (UKCC) produced its *Code of Professional Conduct*, which Burnard and Morrison (1990) suggest is one way of thinking about ethical dilemmas, particularly in relation to research. The UKCC Code states that:

> *Each registered nurse, midwife and health visitor shall act, at all times, in such a manner as to justify public trust and confidence, to uphold and enhance the good standing and reputation of the profession, to serve the interests of society and above all to safeguard the individual patients and clients (UKCC, 1984).*

Intrinsic within all the established codes is the need to respect the client/patient as an individual. Henry (1991) supports Duffy's (1984) view that a major rule in any kind of research is 'respect for persons'. In evoking respect for persons, there is concern for their welfare and respect for the respondents' wishes (Harris, 1985).

One way of considering the ethical responsibilities of the researcher is to examine those available moral codes and guidelines, which go some way towards identifying the researcher's obligations to the respondents of the study, to his/her sponsors and employers and to the development of knowledge.

The identified guidelines are supplemented by specific publications, for example the RCN guidelines on *Confidentiality in Nursing* and the UKCC (1987) *Advisory Paper on Confidentiality*. With all this information available, the researcher has, at least, a starting point from which to plan a research programme which minimises, but does not entirely exclude, the possibility of unethical practice.

Before embarking on any research programme, it is imperative that the researcher has skills specific to that programme. For example, if undertaking interviews, a high level of communication and interpersonal skills are essential. Field and Morse (1985) comment that, in the education of nurses, there is an emphasis on communication skills, so nurse researchers are at an advantage. Nurse education today, with its problem solving approach, should equip qualified nurses with the skills required to carry out research as they 'attempt to extend knowledge through systematic enquiry' (Hockey, 1986). Yet, as with all skills which may be learned, their development is dependent on practice (Cormack, 1984).

Is it enough, though, to be a skilled researcher? Does this in itself automatically lead to ethical behaviour? No code of professional conduct can reflect the personal values of an individual, but only set parameters for the expected behaviour of the individual as a professional. Bias in research programmes can take many forms, either as a result of the researchers personal views, as Henry and Pashley (1990) identify (e.g. a health professional studying the effect of electroconvulsive therapy who objects to it on a personal level) or, as mentioned earlier, because of the pressure of sponsors who may well have expected outcomes. It is also possible for the non-participant observer to influence the way in which respondents respond (Cormack, 1984) and this ultimately puts into question the validity of the research. Therefore, researchers unable to detach themselves must accept personal responsibility for the ethical implications of the process of their research and its subsequent results (Henry and Pashley, 1990).

Assuming the researcher follows implicitly his/her code of professional conduct and is free from prejudice, then the ethical considerations and concerns can be focused realistically. Clarke and Robinson (1989) re-iterate the notion that the researcher may have his/her own moral problems to resolve and must also be aware of the need to adhere to the guidelines of his/her own professional codes and ethical committees as well as perhaps even those of parallel professions.

Ethical committees and codes of practices are designed to aid in the decision-making processes underlying health care research. Their main aim is to monitor research proposals and to safeguard both the patient and the researcher. Members of the ethical committees ought to have an educational background in professional ethics and, therefore, should be well informed of the ethical codes related to research, which must be universally applicable across the health professions (Henry and Pashley, 1990). Given that health care is best delivered through a team approach, ethical codes ought not to be exclusive to one profession, i.e. the medical doctors.

Sheehan (1985) suggests that nursing practice is concerned with enhancing professional knowledge whilst retaining a professional ethic. Although research is necessary to the development of knowledge and understanding in the health care domain, the need to pursue patient care and the protection of patients' rights must also be emphasised. To achieve the latter, constant reflection and critical analysis of health care practice must rest on moral integrity. According to Faulder (1985), an excessive number of patients are being used in clinical trials without their knowledge or consent. The doctors performing these trials justify this action by suggesting that the patients do not understand the scientific reasons underlying the study. With the use of models of care for clients in most health care situations, the involvement of the clients in planning their care is implicit. It would follow then, that, for these clients to be participants in a research project to enhance care, this involvement would continue and the clients would be totally aware of why their treatment was being monitored. Their decision to remain involved would, therefore, be one of informed consent.

Faulder (1985) argues that informed consent involves two issues: first, **the right to know** and, second, **the right to say no**. It is problematic to measure consent and the degree to which it can be considered to be **informed**. Henry (1991) comments that there can be no justification for omitting to tell subjects of their participation in research. However, the question arises as to what we mean by informed consent. What would any of us want to know, in order to make decisions as to whether to participate? The term 'informed consent' is ambiguous and not easy to define or interpret (Henry and Pashley, 1990ii). One way of considering this concept is to acknowledge that it involves respect to the autonomy of all persons. Within informed consent is the implicit respect for persons, whilst still leaving scope for the researcher to evaluate his/her own motives for pursuing a particular line of research. The researcher must remember that implicit within informed consent is the fact that the client must be given sufficient information for an informed choice to be made, recognising the disadvantaged situation and vulnerability of the patient by virtue of being a patient.

The issue of confidentiality has been a matter for discourse in health care for many years. The development of research in nursing has necessitated the inclusion of confidentiality within its planning remit. Baly (1984) refers to the duality of confidentiality in having both moral and legal dimensions. In planning a project, then, the researcher must bear these aspects in mind to ensure that confidentiality is not at risk of being breached. Tschudin (1986) suggests that the notion of confidentiality rests on trust. The RCN (1980) guidelines on confidentiality state that the nurse is in a position of trust and, therefore, must preserve the client's confidences unless relieved of this obligation by lawful excuse. Hence, it is fundamental for the researcher to use his/her interpersonal skills to develop a trusting relationship with prospective participants and allow them to be privy to the research hypothesis. They can then give their informed consent in the knowledge that the researcher has a person and will not breach confidentiality.

An important consideration is that health care may involve studying in detail the work of individual health professionals, who may not be nurses. The researcher may come across compromising situations (e.g. the identification of substandard care or the identification of inadequate resources, but no funds are available to improve the situation). Educationalists may identify curriculum inadequacies (e.g. lack of ethical content), however, a validated curriculum cannot be immediately changed. The researcher needs to have the appropriate skills to deal with the moral dilemmas that may arise as a consequence.

References

American Nurses' Association (ANA) (1968). The nurse in research, ANA guidelines on ethical values, *Amer J Nurs*, **68**, 7, 1304–1307

Baly M (1984). *Professional Responsibility* (2nd edn), John Wiley & Sons, Chichester

Burnard P and Morrison P (1990). *Nursing Research in Action: Developing Basic Skills*, Macmillan, London

Canadian Nurses' Association (1972). Ethics of nursing research, *Canadian Nurse*, **68**, 9, 23–25

Clarke E and Robinson K M (1989). *Nursing Research: Ethics and Methods, Module 6*, South Bank Polytechnic, London

Cormack D F S (1984). *The Research Process in Nursing*, Blackwell Scientific Publications, London

Downie R S and Calman K C (1989). *Healthy Respect: Ethics in Health Care*, Faber & Faber, London

Duffy M E (1985). Designing nursing research: the qualitative quantitative debate, *J Adv Nurs*, **10**, 225–232

Faulder C (1985). *Whose Body is it? The troubling issue of informed consent*, Virago, London

Field P A and Morse J M (1985). *Nursing Research: The Application of Qualitative Approaches*, Croom Helm, London

Harris J (1985). *The Value of Life*, Routledge & Kegan Paul, London

Henry I C and Pashley G (1990). *Health Care Research*, Quay Publishing, Lancaster

Henry I C and Pashley G (1990ii). *Health Care Ethics*, Quay Publishing, Lancaster

Henry I C (1992). Reasonable care: Approaches to health care research, *J Adv Health Nurs Care*, **1**, 4, 79–89

Hockey L (1986). *Nursing Research, Mistakes and Misconceptions*, Churchill Livingstone, Edinburgh

International Council of Nurses (ICN) (1985). *Guidelines for Nursing Research Development*, ICN, Geneva

Royal College of Nursing (RCN) (1977). *Ethics Related to Research in Nursing*, RCN, London

RCN (1980). *Guidelines on Confidentiality in Nursing*, RCN, London

Schrock R (1984). Moral issues in nursing research, Cormack D F S ed, *The Research Process in Nursing*, Blackwell Scientific Publications, London, pp 193–204

Sheehan J (1985). Ethical considerations in nursing practice, *J Adv Nurs*, **10**, 331–336

Tschudin V (1986). *Ethics in Nursing — the Caring Relationship*, Butterworth Heinemann, London

Tschudin V (1989). Ethics, morality and nursing, Hincliff S, Norman S and Schober J eds, *Nursing Practice and Health Care*, Edward Arnold, London, pp 187–202

United Kingdom Central Council for Nursing, Midwifery and Health Visiting (UKCC) (1984). *Code of Professional Conduct for the Nurse, Midwife and Health Visitor* (2nd edn), UKCC, London

Winkler E R (1993). From Kantianism to Contextualism: The Rise and Fall of the Paradigm Theory in Bioethics, in *Applied Ethics: A reader*, Winkler E R and Coombs J R, Blackwells, Oxford pp 333–365.

6

An ethic of care
in nursing research
Kevin Kendrick

'...respect for persons, a central and indispensable normative principle, p391 E W Keyserlingk

The previous chapter introduces major ethical issues, both generally and specifically to nursing research, giving a broad profile of important issues that nurse researchersmust consider from a professional researcher's perspective. This chapter takes some of the specific issues further by extending the debate on the concept of care within the paradygm of research practice that ought to be central for the practitioner researcher in health care. It, clearly, identifies underpinning ethical theory and applies them exceptionally well to real health care research examples.

Introduction

Nursing is in a state of dynamic flux: Project 2000, the higher award and open access to higher education illustrates the academic developments which are steering the profession towards the millenium. This, coupled with innovative advances in the clinical areas nursing development units, clinical practice development units and the named nurse concept all bear testimony to the progressive nature of contemporary practice.

Underpinning all of these themes is the language of professionalism; nurses are charged with the tenets of accountable and responsible practice. A necessary element for achieving these obligations is to place nursing on a rich and well-informed research base (Kendrick 1992). However, research, by its very nature, demands ethical insight and understanding. This chapter will explore the moral dimensions of nursing research and trace the ethical issues involved in the expansion of knowledge.

Guiding principles

Research is essentially concerned with a search for truth — but this can be an arduous endeavour as Kendrick and Kinsella (1993) comment:

> *'the truth is often hidden behind a veil of secrecy and mystique — lifting it can create both light and shadow".*

It is at the interface between 'light and shadow' that moral awareness is needed most.

Nursing research needs to have an ultimate aim and focus; Clarke (1991:22) gives some direction on this issue:

> *'Nursing is essentially a practice-based discipline which involves human interaction. As a result, nursing research is orientated towards the improvement of such practices with human beings'.*

Emerging from this is a clear imperative that the ethos of caring, so central to nursing, must not be compromised or exploited during the research process. Ethics cannot give simple answers to moral questions arising within research — but it can provide certain principles which, when enacted, preserve the dignity and respect of all those involved with it.

There are certain fundamental maxims on which ethical analysis and debate can be focused. Faulder (1985) lists five key principles as being particularly important during the research process, namely:

■ Autonomy
■ Respect for persons
■ Veracity (truthfulness)
■ Beneficence (to do good)
■ Non-maleficence (to do no harm)

All of these principles are interlinked with each other and form the foundations on which relationships should be based in health care. Each deserves individual consideration although a unifying theme draws them all together — the notion of duty.

Duties, imperatives and moral laws

Kant believed that there were absolute moral principles which could never be violated. Indeed, the ability to recognise and act upon these maxims was, for Kant, a central aspect of expressing human rationality. Emerging from this thinking was a series of complex moral rules which are known as the **Categorical Imperative**. Each part of the imperative is interlinked to the next and reflects the absolute nature of Kant's moral stance. The first formulation of the imperative may be simplified in the following way:

■ An action is only moral if you are willing for it to be applied to everyone, yourself included, as a universal law.

The essence of this part of the imperative is concerned with the belief that all people are worthy of equal respect. It asks us all, as commensurate moral agents, never to undertake and action against others which we are not willing to have taken against ourselves. Such a moral tenet clearly reflects the Judaeo–Christian theme of 'do unto others as you would like done unto yourself'. An essential and interesting premise emerges from this for the process of research; the nature and purpose of the research should be as acceptable to the people conducting the enquiry as if they were subjects within the research process. This is vitally important; it ensures that individuals remain valued subjects with intrinsic worth and value not reduced to the devalued status of objects in the cours of research. Quite simply, researchers have no mandate on which to ask people to be part of a research process if they could not honestly and willingly also agree to be a part of that process. Whilst such an acknowledgement could not usually be enacted in a 'real' situation — it bears testimony to the ethical nature and standards of both the researchers and their method.

The second part of Kant's Categorical Imperative builds upon the first formulation and may be simplified in the following way:

■ For an action to be moral, it must never lead to people being seen as 'means to an end' but always as 'ends' in their own right.

In this formulation, Kant is making a clear stand against any form of practice which uses people solely as 'means to an end'. So often in research, the direction of progress, the importance of results and even the limitations of time can lead to participants being used as 'stepping stones' in the research process. The individual concerns and goodwill of subjects become immersed in the freneticism of research as quantitative indicators prevail over the subjective elements of those who have taken part. All of this can escalate to the point where the wellbeing of the research programme takes precedent over that of individual subjects. This is especially so in cases where the research may lead to very beneficient outcomes. Take the hypothetical position that a certain form of clinical research would lead to a universal panacea against cancer — with a small proviso, a small but significant number of mortalities would occur. If we could obtain such a wonderful end through research — would some deaths not be acceptable given the great amount of good which would be generated for humankind? (Utilitarians would argue that fatalities of this nature would be valid given the amount of goodness it would mean for the vast majority of people — but more of this later). Kantian ethics would almost certainly denounce such research as moral anathema; people can never be sacrificed for the greater good because all people are of equal worth, therefore it is impossible to differentiate between individuals for the greater wellbeing of a group even if the benefits for that group were quite startling.

The third and final part of the Categorical Imperative may be expressed in the following, simplified way:

■ In wishing to be moral, individuals must act as members of a community where everybody is seen as having intrinsic worth (ends in their own right).

The central theme in this final formulation is that all individuals share equal parity and worth in moral decision-making; it ensures that nobody can claim moral ascendency within the community. Kant intended this to mean that people should acknowledge and respect the freedom of other individuals to hold moral perspectives and to act upon them. A basic element of human interaction is that we encounter other individuals who hold different perspectives to our own. Kendrick (1993) comments upon this theme by stating:

'Whilst it is legitimate to hold contradicting attitudes towards the same issue, the central principle is that both parties have equal licence to hold, express and defend their respective positions'.

If the tenets of the third formulation of the Categorical Imperative are applied to research, it demands that the person conducting the research is free from any negative bias towards those participating. This can be illustrated by considering the hypothetical example of somebody who is involved with research into HIV or AIDS. It may be that this person comes into contact with drug users and gay men during the course of the work and the notion of a lifestyle which is either gay or drug dependent may be anathema to the researcher. Irrespective of personal subjectivity, the individual must accept that other people have licence to live in a way which is at variance with dominant norms and values, but this does not permit the enactment of prejudice within the research process, either through word or deed — as Norton (1975), paraphrasing Nightingale, states :

the first duty of the researcher is that the research shall do the participant no harm'.

This brief resume of Kant's Categorical Imperative reflects an approach towards moral enquiry which is based upon the motivational factors influencing actions rather than their consequences or outcomes. Nursing has traditionally adopted a very strong relationship with the notion of duty — it is the foundation on which the delivery of care has been conventionally based. The essence of duty is given focus and direction by the five principles which were mentioned earlier, namely: autonomy, respect for persons, veracity, beneficence, non-maleficence. Each of these maxims will now be addressed in relation to the research process.

Autonomy

In its most basic form, autonomy simply means 'self-governing'. However, the manner in which this is enacted, the process of governance, is a complex process which demands harmony and interdependence in the realm of human relationships. It is facile to talk of autonomy in its abstract form; such a theme would demand social isolation akin to the single survivor of a shipwreck, marooned on a desert island, only then could one truly be self-governing. Society relies upon human commerce and interaction to give it form and solidarity. If each member of society were to suddenly cease communications and encounters with other individuals then the very fabric of society would crumble. Even those individuals who seek the contemplative life of a hermit need to interface with the broader society because total self-subsistence is, to all intents and purposes, impossible in the modern age.

Although it is impossible to envisage a state of pure individual autonomy being enacted, this does not mean that we cannot strive to facilitate the expression of and respect for other individual's governance. In this way, self-government is based upon the reciprocal theme that all people may expect to have their autonomy respected and to mirror the same consideration for others.

One of the most important elements for both creating and respecting a person's right to self-government, as a participant in the research process, is to obtain an informed consent. Raanan Gillon, both a doctor and a philosopher, describes the central essence of consent as:

> *'a voluntary, uncoerced decision, made by a sufficiently competent or autonomous person on the basis of adequate information and deliberation, to accept rather than reject*

some proposed course of action that will affect him or her.
Consent in this sense requires action by an autonomous agent
based on adequate information and is by definition informed
consent'. Gillon (1986, p113).

In essence, this interpretation of consent, when applied to the
research process, demands that participants maintain their
rights to dignity and control, together with being given as much
information about the research as possible. Of course, the
nature and parameters of research sometimes make it
impossible to give as much detail as we would like. Often, we
are dealing with unknown features and elements which makes
it inconceivable to think of giving an absolute and definitive
statement about all possible outcomes and ramifications.
However, despite these limitations, it is vital to ethical research
that all subjects within the research process are treated with
respect — seeking their informed consent enacts this
consideration and maintains the concept of care for those who
have agreed to give their participative co-operation for
beneficent themes.

Seeking to preserve a person's autonomy through
informed consent is linked to two closely related but quite
different, duty-based principles:

■ beneficence — to do good

■ non-maleficence — to do no harm

As nurses, we can clearly identify with the direction of these
two principles; we wish to do patients only good and to be
proactive in ensuring that no harm comes to them. However,
the relationship between these two principles is a precarious
one. If we spend a moment reflecting upon practice, it
becomes readily apparent that many of the common nursing
actions, whilst having the overall aim of being therapeutic, can
cause a degree of harm. Think of the simple example of an
intramuscular injection — introducing the syringe into muscle
certainly produces some harm (pain). However, the
therapeutic worth of the drug, hopefully, outweighs the initial
trauma of the injection.

This precarious balance between beneficence and non-maleficence can be easily translated to the the themes of research. If the people involved as participants are to succumb to more harm than good then the moral basis for proceeding is completely debased. As with informed consent, it may not be possible to anticipate the harm which may occur during the research process. However, every endeavour and rigorous precaution should be taken to limit the risk and chance of participants being harmed during the research. All of this demands an air of openness and honesty between the researchers and those who are being researched. This takes us on to the principle of truthfulness which is so important to all human interaction and of particular relevance to the research process.

Veracity

At first sight, the concept of truth seems easy to understnad and evokes associations with other similar themes such as honesty, frankness and a sense of the absolute. However, trying to seek the central essence and clarification about what constitutes the 'truth' is fraught with conceptual difficulties. Kendrick and Kinsella (1993) draw clear moral distinctions between lying and making a mistake:

> '*Of central importance during any encounter is the intention and focus of the people involved as to whether they are truthful or seek to deceive. Sometimes, people inadvertantly convey the wrong information which is a mistake; this is morally incompatible with lying as there are major differences between the essence and elements of the two concepts; lying involves the delivery of an intentionally false statement, whereas a mistake lacks the intent to deceive*'.

What emerges from this is that 'truth', in its purest form, is quite ethereal and unobtainable to the human condition. Put simply, trying to mingle truth within the boundaries of human encounters seeks to place perfection within imperfect boundaries. Individuals, by nature, are imperfect; truth, by its very essence, is perfect — the two forms are not compatible. However, whilst we may not be able to attain the elevated heights of absolute truth, this does not prevent us from seeking honesty. This means that we convey the elements of a situation which are **thought** to be accurate. It may be that we unwittingly give information which is wrong, but this is a mistake not a lie.

Honesty and truthfulness are central tenets in the research process; most participants take part in research believing that they can trust those who are conducting the process. This trust forms the central dynamic in the relationship between researchers and subjects; if anything happens to violate this trust, it assaults and destroys the foundations on which the relationship is based. Trust defiled engenders mistrust and almost inevitably, can never be rebuilt.

Faulder (1985) fires a warning shot across our moral bows about the consequences of dealing in dishonesty and breaking trust:

> '*A trust is broken when one party to the relationship deceives the other in some way, irrespective of whether the deceived party discovers the deception. But, of course, if we do catch out the trusted person in a lie, then our sense of outrage is acute. We feel we have been duped, manipulated and coerced; we have been deprived of information; we have possibly made choices which we would not have made had we been fully aware of the facts, or worse still, we have been deprived of choice altogether*'. ....*Faulder (1985, p26)*.

People who agree to take part, as subjects, in the research process are responding to a tacit appeal by the researcher to be trusting. In terms of any form of reciprocation, it seems that the very least a person can expect in return is that this trust is not violated. Endeavouring to be informative, open and honest with clients/patients or colleagues goes a long way towards protecting the trust which is placed within the researcher's gift.

Respect for persons

If a research team seeks to enable the subject's autonomy, gains an informed consent on the grounds of veracity and, maintains a beneficent theme throughout, then it fulfils most, if not all, of the moral criteria inherent within Kant's Categorical Imperative. Indeed, it also means that the research is versed in the meaning and essence of an ethical concept, know as 'respect for persons'. (cf Henry and Pashley, 1990).

This principle has particular relevance to the ethical parameters surrounding research on human subjects. It carries with it the notion that persons have intrinsic worth and value; this does not have to be supported, argued or quantitated. Individuals are, as of nature, worthy of regard and consideration — '*Ris ipsa locquitur*'.

To this point, we have considered a duty-based approach to research. This has been principally applied to nursing but is relevant to any research involving human beings (or any creature for that matter). The themes which have been addressed are Kantian and reflect the ethos of a deontological approach to moral reasoning. During this century, a number of codes have been created to try and protect the rights of subjects during research and provide clear indicators for the preservation of the participant's best interests.

Protective codes

The existence of professional codes helps to promote beneficent themes in practice settings. Burnard and Chapman (1985) expand upon this by arguing that such codes engender confidence amongst clients, the public and society about the direction and focus of the profession — ultimately, codes exist to protect the best interests of those who use or need the services of that profession.

During this century, codes have come into being which present maxims designed to prevent the exploitation of human subjects during research. For example the Nuremberg Code (1945) and the Helsinki Declaration (1957). Both codes share a common ethos which emphasises the obligation upon researchers to respect and uphold the rights of people during research. Beauchamp and Childress (1983, p338) point to informed consent as being a central feature of agreement between researchers and subjects:

'The voluntary consent of the human subject is absolutely essential. This means that the person involved should have legal capacity to give consent; should be so situated as to be able to exercise free power of choice, without the intervention of any element of force, fraud, deceit, duress, over-reaching or other ulterior form of constraint or coercion; and should have sufficient knowledge and comprehension of the elements of the subject matter involved as to enable him to make an understanding and enlightened decision'.

The Nuremberg Code emphatically supports the notion of informed consent by subjects — indeed, that this should be a pre-requisite to any participation within the research process. This clearly reflects a care for individual rights at the epicentre of considerations underpinning the ethics of research. However, not all approaches to moral reasoning place duties as the overriding theme on which actions should be based. A school of ethical analysis called Utilitarianism would argue that the wellbeing of an individual is of secondary importance to that of the 'group'. Utilitarianism has enjoyed tremendous success as a method for moral deliberation — a resumé of its fundamental elements is vital to any discussion involving research on persons.

Research for the greater good

Unlike deontology, utilitarianism argues that actions are morally right when they result in happiness or pleasure for the majority of people. Conversely, an action could be said to be immoral if it failed to secure happiness for the majority. This approach seems to be versed very much in the pragmatic. After all, it would be impossible to please every single individual with each action. However, closer analysis reveals a number of pertinent problems with utilitarianism, and raises some important questions as to its suitability for helping to consider moral issues in the research process.

A fundamental difficulty with utilitarianism is that it seeks to promote happiness for the majority of people — but what is happiness? One person may feel that a cottage in the country would be absolute Utopia whilst another person would feel alienated and miserable away from the frenetic nature of city life. This bears testimony to the notion that a consensus about what constitutes happiness must be achieved before it can be promoted for the majority. Moreover, even when agreement has been reached about the nature of happiness, there is no guarantee that an action will promote it. Utilitarianism cannot predict the outcome of an action and crystal ball gazing is a poor basis on which to conduct moral analysis!

However, there are deeper and more vital issues at stake. Emanating from the problems surrounding the theoretical underpinnings of utilitarianism are fundamental questions about justice and fairness. If we accept a system of morality which seeks to generate happiness for the majority then it means that the minority must be willing to sacrifice their individual wellbeing and interests. When such a method is enacted, it leads to the loss of central ethical themes; if justice is to have depth and relevance then it must be applied to all persons equally. If the minority surrender their interests in favour of the majority, they no longer sit under the umbrella of justice and become subsumed in an equation which promotes the theme of a 'might is right'. In terms of logical progression, such a dynamic also destroys the concept of fairness because, quite simply, how can it be fair that a minority of people can be placed under a position of possible tyranny by the majority? Finally, to talk of rights is quite facile within a utilitarian framework. In such a system, the rights of individuals are dissolved in a swirling vortex of majority consensus. This can have far reaching repercussions. When rights exist and are acknowledged, it places a clear and undeniable obligation upon members of society to uphold and respect them. This has particular impact and relevance to the research process.

Returning to the earlier position that a universal panacea had been found to combat cancer and needed to be researched through clinical trials before it could be marketed. Once again, it is thought that the aggressive nature of drugs would, almost inevitably, lead to some fatalities. However, from a utilitarian perspective, this would be quite acceptable because of the overwhelming amount of happiness it would produce for the present and future generations. Clearly, such a ratio of beneficence outcomes would validate some deaths. Indeed, if the trials are needed before the drug can be widely implemented, then in terms of consequences, a number of fatalities would be wholly acceptable. This demonstrates the death of individual rights when the overriding goal of group happiness becomes of paramount importance. While this example of subjects dying during research is deliberately extreme, it serves to highlight and illustrate the many problematical areas surrounding utilitarianism as a method of ethical analysis in research.

Placing limits on research

This chapter has been concerned with an investigation of those ethical principles which inform ethical standards in research. The themes covered can apply to all research involving human subjects; indeed, they can be applied with equal efficacy to all human encounters and interactions.

As nurses, we have an obligation to place our practice upon the firm footing of rigorous and thorough research. This is vital if nursing is to become an autonomous, accountable and responsible profession. However, in seeking this end, we must ensure that the research we conduct, or are privy to, reflects an ethic of caring — as Faulder (1985, p106) so eloquently states:

'Their trust must not be abused, nor their altruism. These human and moral considerations are more important than

any scientific advance, and it is these obligations which impose the limits to science'.

References

Beauchamp T L (1983). *Principles of biomedical ethics*, Oxford University Press, Oxford, p338.

Burnard P and Chapman C M (1985). *Professional and ethical issues in nursing*, John Wiley and Sons, Chichester.

Clarke J (1991). Moral dilemmas in nursing research. Nursing Practice, **4**, 4, 22.

Faulder C (1985). *Whose body is it? The troubling issue of informed consent*, Virago Press, London, p26.

Faulder C (1985). *Whose body is it? The troubling issue of informed consent*, Virago Press, London, p106.

Gillon R (1986). *Philosophical medical ethics*, John Wiley and Sons, Chichester, p113.

Henry C and Pashley G (1990). *Health Ethics*, Quay Publishing, Lancaster.

Kendrick K D (1992). considerations of personhood in nursing research: an ethical perspective, in Soothill K, Henry I C and Kendrick K D, *Themes and perspectives in nursing*, Chapman and Hall, London.

Kendrick K D (1993). Not just for ivory towers – Ethics at the interface, *Brit J Nurs* (in press).

Kendrick K D (1993). 'Lifting the veil' – truth telling in palliative care, *Intnl J Cancer Care* (in press).

Keyserlingk E W (1993). Ethics Codes and Guidelines for Health Care and Research: Can Respect for Autonomy be a Multiculture Principle? in Winkler E R and Coombs J R, *Applied Ethics: A reader*, Blackwell, Oxford.

Norton D (1975). The research ethic, *Nurs Times*, **71**, 52, 2048–2049.

7

Informed consent
In therapeutic practice and research
Norma Fryer

'I became silent, and this struck the others silent too. I could see they were bewildered and all the comfort of their travels was gone....'C S Lewis, p257.

The previous chapter examined the underpinning ethical theory related to research practice, whereas this chapter debates the concept of 'Informed Consent' itself. This is seen as essential for good ethical research practice. Not only does it deal with central ethical issues of informed consent but there is an important discussion on aspects of therapeutic and non-therapeutic practice within the health care field.

This chapter will examine informed consent in relation to the patient as an autonomous agent within the decision-making processes involved in both the sphere of therapeutic practice and health care research. The intention is to identify the professional and moral implications of obtaining consent from the perspective that the patient has a personal responsibility, implicit in the principle of autonomy, to actively participate in the decision-making process, where those decisions directly effect the health and wellbeing of the individual concerned.

The concept of 'informed consent' is central to both the processes of therapeutic practice and to clinical research and cannot be divorced from addressing any issue involving patients. It is equally important to acknowledge the notion of personal autonomy for both patient and practitioner as an underpinning moral principle of respect for persons. As such, respect for the person and for the autonomy of that person becomes a major feature in both the therapeutic relationship and in the choices and decisions made by both parties. It is clear that, if there is to be a satisfying outcome for both patient and practitioner/researcher, there should be an obligation for information to be exchanged within a climate of mutual respect and trust. As Faulder (1985) so rightly suggests, 'if the doctor does not confide in the patient as the patient confides in the doctor, then the relationship is unequal and unjust' (p 27). In exploring the moral dilemmas faced by health care professionals, and in particular that of the doctor, the unequal relationship between professional and patient will serve to demonstrate the difficulties experienced by many, if not most, patients, in taking responsibility for decisions regarding their own health matters, where personal autonomy is often compromised. This is readily seen when the issue of consent for either therapeutic treatment or participation in research is considered. However, before such an examination, it is important to attempt to unravel the meaning of informed consent and the complexity of its implications in practice.

Consent in health care — background

In examining the meaning of 'informed consent', it is necessary to look first at the background to consent as a principle within health care. As a moral phenomena, it has a very recent place in therapeutic practice and research, with changes in terms of medical practice arising mainly from law. Codes of practice within medicine did not identify the patient's position, other than as the recipient of treatment and care, expressed as a principle of beneficence. The Hippocratic Oath provided the first set of rules to guide physicians in their practice:

> *I will follow that system or regime which, according to my ability and judgement, I consider for the benefit of my patients, and abstain from whatever is deleterious or mischievous (Downie and Calman, 1987, p 246)*

Nowhere in this oath does the judgement or ability of the patient feature as a consideration, emphasising the power and autonomy of the doctor and the paternalism inherent in today's practice of medicine.

The traditions of the Hippocratic Oath have lived on for centuries, serving as a professional and moral code for doctors, with subsequent codes of practice, placing greater emphasis on the health of the patient and a respect for human life. The World Health Organisation's (1968) *Declaration of Geneva* provides such an example, 'I will practice my profession with conscience and dignity; the health of my patient will be my first consideration.'

Once again, there is no reference to the patient's participation and/or an implied or explicit moral responsibility to obtain consent or to be involved in decisions relating to therapeutic practice or research. The absence of such statements can also be noted in the *Code of Professional Conduct for the Nurse, Midwife and Health Visitor* (UKCC, 1984), despite its reference to the importance of the patient's own customs, values and spiritual beliefs.

The most significant move towards the principle of consent resulted from the 'medical' research carried out on humans in Nazi Germany. The atrocities and moral exploitation of humans during this period led to the explicit demands of the *Nuremburg Code*, relating to medical research, including an expressed principle that 'the voluntary consent of the human subject is absolutely essential' (Beauchamp and Childress, 1979, p 287). To support and enhance the principles of this code of practice, further ethical issues were identified within the *Declaration of Helsinki* (1975), which attempted to draw together a balance between the autonomy of the patient as a research subject and the utilitarian principle of the benefits to others. In doing so, a basic principle was drawn up stating that '...concern for the interest of the subject... must prevail over the interest of science and society' (Beauchamp and Childress, 1979, p289).

However, as Beck (1990) points out, included in the same document is a statement which does not support the autonomy of the patient or research subject in that it declares that 'if the doctor consider it essential not to obtain informed consent, the specific reason should be stated on the experimental protocol' (Beck, 1990, p 113). Whilst the notion of informed consent is introduced here, the ethical significance will be discussed once the meaning of 'informed consent' has been explored. Meanwhile, it is suffice to say that, as a concept within health care, 'consent' on its own provides little more than a written or verbal statement indicating that an individual has agreed to a specific course of action. The traditional 'consent forms' signed by patients prior to surgical intervention with an anaesthetic are a good example of the type of consent given, where many patients 'consent' to 'the operation' without appropriate or adequate information being given. Equally common are examples of verbal consent being given for particular procedures to be carried out where patients are not informed of the investigations to be carried out from such procedures.

One of the features of obtaining consent is that it provides the doctor or researcher with evidence that a patient has agreed to a course of action, particularly if the patient has supported the agreement with a signed declaration. However, it is also important to recognise that a state of ill health renders many patients vulnerable, with personal autonomy diminished or removed. In many ways, patients become targets for coercion and exploitation. It is on the basis of this, intentional or otherwise, that the principle of 'informed consent' must be considered as a moral prerogative for all those involved in either therapeutic practice or research.

If a patient is to be respected, expected to act as an autonomous entity (responsible in part for his/her health and maintenance of wellbeing) and not to be subjected to the immorality of coercion/exploitation, it is essential that the therapeutic relationship enhances disclosure from both practitioner and patient (or subject in research practice), rather than disclosure solely from the latter. It is at this point that the meaning of informed consent must be clarified.

Informed consent

The Dictionary of Medical Ethics' definition of informed consent is cited by Gillon (1991) as the:

> ...*voluntary, uncoerced decision made by a sufficiently competent or autonomous person on the basis of information*

> *and deliberation to accept rather than reject some proposed*
> *course of action (p 113).*

The significance of this statement relates to the understanding and application of consent being given by a person who has the capacity to make an informed decision and deliberate choice from an adequate source of information.

The main ethical argument and considerations that informed consent imposes onto the professional in both therapeutic practice and research, centres on the problem of disclosure of information: how much does the patient want to know; how much does the patient need to know and, from a moral perspective, how much information should the patient be given in order to make an informed decision? Whilst the responsibility for this often seems, in practice, to be focused on the professional(s) involved, there is a strong argument to suggest that, for the 'competent' patient (i.e. a person with a capacity for self-determination), such a responsibility should be shared. As Faulder (1985) reminds us:

> *...informed consent is a matter of ethical principle, not a legal*
> *formula or a courtesy which the doctor may or may not*
> *extend to his patients as he thinks fit and only to those he*
> *deems capable of acting upon it... the decision whether to give*
> *or to refuse informed consent always rests with the patient*
> *(p 15).*

If there is to be any acknowledgement of and respect for both the patient's and the practitioner's/researcher's autonomy in matters relating to therapeutic practice or research, it would appear that both or all parties involved should respect the moral obligations they share with each other. To enable both professional and moral judgements to be made, that safeguard the integrity of the patient and the professional, there must be a relationship which encourages a partnership of mutual trust and respect. This can be best identified by examining the situations that may arise in both therapeutic practice and research. However, as Henry and Pashley (1990) clearly state, an important point regarding the concept of consent is that it relates not only to the specific areas of therapeutic practice and research, but to any setting where there is a relationship between patient or client and the health care professional.

Informed consent in therapeutic practice

In addressing the moral arguments affecting therapeutic practice and informed consent, many of the major ethical issues apply equally to the practice of research within health care.

For the purposes of this discussion, particular reference will be made to the doctor, although the principles apply to any therapeutic relationship.

The relationship that exists between the patient and doctor in many areas of medical practice has evolved as one that, through socialisation and greater knowledge, places the doctor in a much stronger and more powerful position than the patient. One of the most significant effects of this process is seen through the paternalistic approach that many doctors have towards their patients; one which is acknowledged and accepted by many patients, whilst others expect nothing less, based on a belief that 'the doctor knows best'. In short:

> ...*paternalism holds that the health professionals should take a parental role towards patients and their families, that they have superior knowledge of medicine and that they alone have a right to decide what is best for patients and their families because of their long and specialised training (Henry and Pashley, 1990, p 31).*

It may be noted that the doctor or nurse, because of his/her specialised training, is also in an 'expert position' as a research and, therefore, 'knows best'.

The position the doctor places himself in and/or is expected to fulfil in therapeutic practice may prove, in many situations, to be one that serves the needs of both patient and practitioner. Professional or moral dilemmas may never arise; the doctor's judgement may turn out to be correct; the patient happy with the outcome of the treatment, knowing no more about how and why specific decisions were made, but satisfied that he/she is 'cured'.

However, whilst there are many patients who do not question the paternalistic role of the doctor, there are many who do. These patients recognise not only the risks of this sort of patient dependency, which has sometimes resulted in 'dehumanisation' (Thiroux, 1980), but also the fact that this dependency diminishes personal autonomy at a time when a person is at his/her most vulnerable and compliant to rational persuasion (Harris, 1991).

A person for whom health is compromised is often in a position where personal autonomy is threatened to some degree, either because of the physical effects of the illness or from the fear associated with even a minor ailment. Hospitalisation adds to the problem, often leaving the patient in a position where any decision he/she may wish to make will depend on, or be influenced by, the relationship with those providing the information and administering the care and treatment. (The person may also be asked to be involved in research.)

In order for patients to be able to make informed decisions and to take responsibility for their participation in their own recovery, optimum wellbeing and/or preparation for death, much will depend on the information given by the doctor or other professionals and the way in which this information is perceived and understood.

It is often suggested that patients, given that they have a right to make an informed choice, will be overwhelmed with information that they may not fully understand. As a consequence, patients may be unnecessarily alarmed at either their diagnosis, their prognosis, or the possible risks of a proposed course of treatment and may find themselves unable to make a decision through confusion and/or fear. The dilemma in practice is very real, as there are some patients who do not understand the technicalities, some who do not wish for that level of information and others who, given that they have the information and understood both the meaning and the implications, choose to act upon the advice of the professional.

(It is in relation to this latter point that the professional, as both practitioner and researcher, is in a position to display empathy rather than an overriding display of paternalism.)

Experience or knowledge of a patient and his/her family may show that some patients may not wish to be involved in the decision-making process and that their view that 'the doctor knows best' is a major part of their own capacity to deal with their illness and/or prognosis. It is difficult, therefore, to follow an absolute principle that all patients must be given all information in the same way. For example, one patient may clearly indicate that he/she wishes to know statistical chances of survival after two years of treatment, so that choice can be made based on how that person can best cope with the likely consequences. Another patient may trust implicitly in the doctor and wish to follow the advice or preference of that doctor. The ethical question here must be, 'Does the patient have a right to remain in ignorance?' Harris (1991) approaches the question by suggesting that, whilst there are many unpleasant things in life that we may not wish to know about, it does not follow that anyone infringes our rights if they inform us. Again, we are left with the question of what we should do.

It would seem that, if we are to respect the autonomy of the person and acknowledge the responsibility of the person for his/her own decisions in relation to his/her health and wellbeing, then any justification for non-disclosure (whether related to a therapeutic decision, participation in research or a decision about prognosis/diagnosis) may only be considered on moral grounds when the patient has expressed a wish to not be given details of the state of his/her health. Given this situation, the health professional would then have to determine what, and how much, information to give. However, this scenario still does not give the patient a 'right' to remain in ignorance.

It is at this point that the position of the 'incompetent' patient should be given some consideration. In the context of health care, this refers to those patients whose autonomy is diminished or absent either through mental impairment, through being in a transient or permanent state of unconsciousness or because the patient is a child. Where weight cannot be given to personal autonomy (i.e. in the cases of those patients who, according to the principles of the Canadian Law Reform Commission (Beauchamp and Childress, 1979), are not able to make reasoned judgement and are not, according to the Commission's standards, 'reasonable people') even greater ethical dilemmas are present.

The first major hurdle lies with the definition of 'incompetence', as there are persons who, whilst being limited in the management of their own affairs, may not be incapable of making autonomous choices, especially if these choices do not harm others. The degree to which a person is considered incompetent, as for example with children or those persons whose illness and its effects renders them transiently incapacitated, does not necessarily imply that they are unable to make what Harris (1991, p 215) refers to as a'maximally autonomous' decision. In fact, Harris suggests that to respect autonomy is to respect a person's decisions made in the light of their present character and priorities. As such, it is difficult to provide parameters when individual judgement is so value-laden.

Examples in case law, in both the UK and the USA, have clearly shown how decisions regarding the sterilisation of mentally impaired young women caused both legal and professional ethical dilemmas, where outcomes have indicated the difficulty of providing any absolute legal or moral law. The existing law in the UK gives no legal rights to relatives within the context of consent to either giving or withholding treatment. Yet, it is within the moral perspective of consent that there appears to be no greater argument for the professional to make decisions for an 'incompetent' patient, than for a relative to make these decisions.

Indeed, it would seem reasonable to suggest that the motives of either relative or professional may be questioned in relation to the principle of beneficence and/or the utilitarian maxim of the greater happiness for the greater number. Where decisions are made for another person, is it possible to determine the greatest benefits for this person? It is at this point that the more specific issue of informed consent in relation to research will be addressed.

Informed consent within health care research

Informed consent within health care research contains many of the ethical dimensions found in the everyday practice of therapeutic care. Yet, it is through the process of carrying out research that many of the issues of informed consent were initially raised. Codes of practice relating to research have already been discussed, highlighting some contradictions and deficiencies in their interpretation and meaning.

Through ethics committees, moral issues are addressed in relation to research within the health care field. Henry and Pashley (1990, p 52) identify these principles, many of which could, and should, be applied to therapeutic practices and care within all health care domains:

- respect for person autonomy
- protection for patients/subjects
- avoidance of fraud, duress and anxiety
- self-audit; identifying motives for suggested treatment/procedures
- promotion of rational decisions by professionals
- promotion of public values

In therapeutic research, it is often easier to recognise the possibility of utilising such principles when the patient, involved with the decision making, is anticipating some direct, personal benefit from his/her participation in the research programme. Whilst it is possible to see how such patients may be coerced and/or exploited for the reasons described earlier, it is within the realms of non-therapeutic research where the more complex issues may arise.

When non-therapeutic research is carried out, where there may be no benefit to the participant, the overriding principle of beneficence is immediately contradicted. Such research, often carried out as a clinical trial must, by law, avoid trespass to the person, which in moral terms means there must be no evidence of violation of the individual's personal autonomy. The Kantian principle of treating people as an end, not merely as a means to an end, is clearly difficult in such a process. Yet, as Gillon (1991) emphasises, there is still a moral argument that, in carrying out non-therapeutic research, the principle of non-maleficence should be respected.

Whilst there may be possible consequences in applied research, in that there may be no guaranteed benefits and a possibility of side effects or minimal risks, there is a moral responsibility to treat research subjects in the same way as patients within the therapeutic relationship, in that all the principles of informed consent apply. Then the participant, with the full knowledge of the possible consequences, will be able to make an informed decision whether to consent to any participation or not.

When the professional is involved in research which uses randomised controlled trials, there are obvious moral dilemmas with respect to the issue of informed consent. Whilst the participants may consent to their involvement, in the knowledge that they may or may not benefit from the drug or treatment used, there are two major moral concerns which neither the patient nor the professional can avoid. First, whilst the professional may be more knowledgeable about the potential of the treatment being tried, the very nature of the exercise means that neither party is in possession of the evidence. Second, where the research process involves a single or double 'blind' trial of a drug, neither the patient in the former case, nor the professional or the patient in the latter situation, will be aware of the actual drugs being used. This is even more so the case when a placebo is used. As such, the nature of the research invalidates informed consent. Botros (1990) goes so far as to claim that if informed consent can make an otherwise impermissible randomised controlled trial permissible, it is to give consent 'a role which goes beyond that which it plays in therapy' (p 19).

Furthermore, whilst the use of placebos within and outside research practices may serve to confirm or exclude possibilities relating to the causes or effects of diseases, there appears to be no moral justification for administering either a placebo or alternative drug, known to be of little therapeutic value in research or therapeutic practice. Harris (1991) argues that the only justification for using drugs in a trial is where there is a genuine uncertainty about which of the two remedies is most effective; therefore, the best treatment will be either of the drugs chosen at random. Equally, it could be argued that whilst there is evidence that patients have benefited from the use of placebos, there appears to be little moral justification to support an action where the patient has consented to treatment based on deception or misleading information. The important issue remains the same. Has the patient been informed?

In addressing the factors that the concept of informed consent highlights, it is clear that the personal autonomy of the patient is central to the underlying moral issues that are presented in both therapeutic practice and research. Whilst the position of the health professional, especially that of the doctor provides a strong and paternalistic element in the decision-making processes involved in health care, it is the patient who is central to the choices that are made.

However, whilst the patient has a major role to play in decision making, where their personal health and wellbeing is concerned, there appears to be evidence in practice that there is often little acknowledgement from the medical profession, particularly although not exclusively, of the patients autonomous nature as a person, especially where '...that would seem to interfere with the expedient benevolence of the practitioner' (Nash, 1990, p 118). Perhaps relinquishing the paternalistic role, the professional would allow the patient to recognise more clearly the personal accountability involved in health care practice. Where personal autonomy, with its inherent notion of personal responsibility and moral principle of respect for persons is valued by both professional and patient, there is a much greater prospect for the patient to appreciate the real implications of being responsible for making choices in health care. The issues surrounding informed consent provide a framework on which all other aspects concerning the patient/professional relationship are built. If we are to see patients as self-determining persons who are able to think about ends and decide on the means by which these ends are fulfilled, it is vital that they are respected as such beings in a state of health or illness. Giving opportunity for choices in giving or withholding consent is clearly 'enhancing' the central principle of respect for persons with health care research and practice.

References

Beauchamp T L and Childress J F (1979). *Principles of Biomedical Ethics*, Oxford University Press, Oxford

Beck P (1990). Informed consent, Evans D ed, *Why should we care?*, Macmillan, London

Botros S (1990). Equipoise, consent and the randomised clinical trials, Byrne P ed, *Ethics and Law in Health Care Research*, John Wiley and Sons, Chichester.

Downie R S and Calman K C (1987). *Healthy Respect — Ethics in Health Care*, Faber and Faber, London.

Faulder C (1985). *Whose Body is it?*, Virago, London

Gillon R (YEAR?). Philosophical Medical Ethics, John Wiley and Sons, Chichester.

Harris J (1991). *The Value of Life*, Routledge and Kegan Paul, London, p 208

Henry C and Pashley G (1990). Health Ethics, Quay Publishing, Lancaster

Lewis C S (1956). *'Till We Have Fairies'* A myth retold, Fount, Harper-Collins, Glasgow.

Nash P (1990). Autonomy, Competence and Mental Disorders, Evans D ed, *Why should we care?*, Macmillan, London.,

Thiroux J P (1980). *Ethics – Theory and Practice*, Glencoe Publishing Co/ Collier Macmillan Publishers, London, p 281

United Kingdom Central Council for Nursing, Midwifery and Health Visiting (UKCC) (1984). *Code of Professional Conduct for the Nurse, Midwife and Health Visitor*, UKCC, London

Section 2

In pursuit of ethical practice in research

8 Ethical boundaries of research
Referring to the concept of the person
Christine Henry

This first chapter of section two introduces the philosophical foundations and ethical issues of good research practice. It attempts to identify the skeletal framework in which to encapsulate the processes of research and forms of applied knowledge, useful for raising levels of awareness in carrying out research in health care practice. Whilst the focus is upon 'persons', it identifies and debates ethical issues concerned with the use of other animals and humans in research. The chapter identifies the major landmarks and attempts to profile the ethical boundaries of research practice, formulating the outline on which to draw the details of the ethical map for good health care research.

Research is concerned with the extension of knowledge. Health care research in particular uses knowledge from a variety of disciplines from within the natural and social science domains, which should involve the person in terms of her/his biology, psychology, social and moral features. Research demands increased understanding of our life world and the physical albeit creative universe in which we have 'being' and is central to education and professional practice. We can relate one idea with another, compare instances, search for patterns, form expectations and make predictions. Understanding and explanation is often encapsulated within boundaries of generalisation. Whilst generalisation may be a common aim for all research it is crucial to acknowledge that different approaches place different levels of emphasis upon the requirement to generalise. The philosophical question underpinning research practice raises the question of how far we can generalise about the person? The term 'person' is not a natural term like homosapien (species specific) and is often viewed as a non-natural concept. It may be useful to discuss persons in relation to the ethical boundaries of research practice, particularly in the health and social fields and consider medical and health care research practice. A focus will be given to the use of other animals and humans in research.

Persons

Henry (1986) remarks that a traditional philosophical view sees the person as essentially a mental being. Psychological and biological facts can provide evidence for personhood but cannot constitute a definition or full explanation of the essence of persons. The person has rationality exercised by thinking and the use of language. These are distinguishing features and are studied and researched through first order cognitive psychological domains. A materialistic view is put forward by Ryle (1949). He rejects Cartesian dualism and claims that the term 'mind' is used as if it referred to an invisible entity inhabiting the body, 'a ghost in the machine'. Ryle's philosophy reflects analytical behaviourism with a person's psychological features viewed as analysable in terms of behaviour. He remarks that both 'idiots' (Ryle's term) and very young infants do not have complicated behaviour or dispositional traits and therefore do not have minds and are not persons. However, the very young infant and mentally disadvantaged may be treated as persons on **moral grounds**. This relates to the principle of valuing them. If this is not a moral principle to follow, then from Ryle's position and in relation to research, both very young infants and the mentally disadvantaged could be viewed as passive subjects / objects for research. The social values, together with being members of a rational species and identifiably human, influence who may be or may not be treated as persons and therefore valued, given rights, responsibility and choice. Having person status prevents individuals from being disregarded in some way. (In research on embryos and in animal experimentation this aspect will be seen to be crucial for the ethical debate). Persons are given rights, value and respect. Central to health care research is respect for persons and most professions have developed codes of conduct or practice that enhance this principle. The British Psychological Society (1991), for example, address issues of relevance to their own research workers and the Code of Conduct for Psychologists opens with the statement:

'In all their work psychologists shall value integrity, impartiality and respect for persons.....'

The British Psychological Society, much like other professions, points out that research should be carried out with the highest standards of scientific integrity and this is only possible if there is mutual respect and confidence between the researcher and the respondents. Good research emphasise scientific integrity and implicit is the right and dignity of participants i.e. the persons. In other words, scientific enquiry is not value- free and 'scientific integrity' involves the central theme of respect for persons.

From a traditional philosophical stance distinguishing features emerge for persons and these have often been used as guidelines in an attempt to distinguish persons from non-persons. However, the present author takes the view that such a criteria for person definitions should not be used, advocating instead, valuing the whole person, not particular parts or features. Features such as reason, language and intelligence emphasise that mind is a central feature of persons in the traditional sense. This feature list or traditional view develops into an image of an ideal or formalised conception of persons mirrored through Dennett's (1979) model of necessary but not sufficient, conditions. Persons are rational beings who have special psychological intentional states. A social feature is that persons are objects of a particular stance and should be treated as persons, and therefore capable of reciprocating in some way. Being self conscious is a condition of persons being capable of becoming moral agents. However, being an agent who is self conscious allows for valuing one's self and others, being 'other regarding' and capable of having moral values, reflecting and making moral judgements.

Abelson (1977) builds upon the social and moral aspects and claims that the term 'person' is evaluative (valued) and not open to biological or empirical analysis. A person is a subject of both psychological and moral traits. According to Abelson it is possible to give 'person status' to a non-human. The alien ET, the chimpanzee and the dolphin are like us in some ways and therefore ascription of person status to these may be meaningfully applied. The term person is evaluative and can be seen to be a moral concept like the term 'good'. Social values and ideologies will also influence the ascription of person status. We are all aware through social history of how a race of people was stripped of person status in Nazi Germany. Some individuals clearly give semi-person status to the severely mentally retarded or madly insane whilst others will ascribe person status to the embryo, dolphin, pet dog or cat and even the goldfish. A crucial point lies with this ascription of person status because rights and respect are necessarily attributed to the individual. This is the focal point of why the person and the potential person argument was not appropriate for the debate on embryonic research and why conflicts arise in relation to animal rights. (Animals are used in research). Whilst some animals would clearly not make it into the person class, the argument surrounds the moral issues of ascribing rights of some kind on their behalf by persons who, by their own status, have the potential for 'moral integrity'. This raises an important question, particularly for medical research. Should it be only persons for whom rights and respect are considered within research practice? Warnock (1985) remarks that the special status of the human embryo and its protection by law does not depend upon when it becomes as person. This relates to the notion that we cannot give an answer to the question of when and at what stage of development the developing human becomes a person; if full status is given to the early embryo such ascription demands the rights and legal entactments properly accorded to persons. The Warnock report does not identify the status of the embryo. The only reference to the status of the embryo is a demand for more respect than other animal subjects. Nevertheless, it causes concern when other animal subjects used in experimentation have no status or rights at all. In this sense the term status is used in an evaluative way. It also clearly objectifies other animals; if other animals have no rights their status is equivalent to a 'thing', an object to be used in research practice. In a descriptive sense their status may be at a low level in that they are treated as objects. According to Warnock the embryo is not a person and may be viewed as a collection of cells; it is only on implantation that the embryo has potential to become a person.

Once again there is the principle placed upon value given to the embryo and other animals. The parents who have conceived will give a value to the fertilised ovum, and through that 'value' recognise the potential for 'personhood'. This may occur even at the early stages of embryonic development. The value of a 'potential child' has moral and social status. The value principle is very different from the biological or factual description of a collection of cells. Furthermore, a relationship between the growing embryo and the parents develops. The social relationship will influence the idea of how we conceptualise and subsequently treat the embryo or the six month old foetus. We may clearly conceptualise the embryo as a person to ourselves. Similarly, it may be the way in which we 'personify' our pet dog, cat or goldfish.

So far we have the feature list or the traditional model for distinguishing between persons and non-persons and Abelson's evaluative model. Both models raise ethical issues in medical or health care research.

The commonsense model of persons takes the social aspects as central. Teichman(1972) remarks that everyday use of language within the social context is important. The terms 'human' and 'person' are viewed as identical. In philosophical terms, they are not identical, i.e. the term 'person' is normative and evaluative, whereas the term human is semi-normative, referring to things we value in being human and descriptive in the sense of being a member of a species. The social context is crucial. In our language games, meaning is in how we use a term, therefore we use the term 'human' to mean the same as the 'person'. Natural persons, unlike artificial persons, (i.e. the thinking machine, cf next section) have living bodies recognised as belonging to the human species. This notion of having a particular body that is recognisably human excludes parrots (who talk), dolphins and chimpanzees, although some research shows that they have similar features to persons in that they may well have conceptual thought and can communicate in their own way.

The important aspect of this model is upon the everyday functions of language associated with a 'commonsense' view of the world. 'Human' is a starting point for understanding and identifying persons, particularly from our own perspective.

The author's exploratory study in 1985 was partly concerned with 'commonsense' conceptions of the nature of persons. Specific attention was paid to person and non-person distinctions and also features of the person. Results indicated from a cohort of 84 respondents that there was a development trend in 'person', 'non-person' distinctions. Young children gave rather concrete and materialistic conceptions, in that there was no distinction evident between the terms 'human' and 'person'. This indicated that the children were influenced by their social experience and social context meaning in use. Older respondents and adults (nurses, doctors and teachers) gave more rational and dualistic conceptions of persons, emphasising the mind as being a central feature of persons. They tended to refer to a more traditional and formal conception of persons. (i.e. the feature list proposed by philosophers such as Dennett).

What does this mean in relation to research practice? Indirectly, it may indicate that, generally, we have a tendency to formally conceptualise persons in the traditional way (cf Dennett's model). The feature list encourages us to distinguish between persons and non-persons. If children view the term as equating to human and adults conceptualise persons by a traditional model, then we may therefore assume that:

■   Persons must give their consent if they are to be involved in any research project and we should recognise their autonomy and therefore accord them respect. However, it may give us licence to mask the 'value' and respect accorded to other 'non-humans' or non-persons, other animals and use them as objects in research. The conclusion is made that if they do not have person features, then they have no value, status or respect - (note Nazi Germany).

■   It may be much more appropriate to take Abelson's model of 'persons', in that it is a moral term like the term 'good'. Furthermore, it is open to us to whom we prescribe person status. Neither biological, behavioural or psychological traits will determine for us who should and should not be counted as a person.

Person and Non-Person Distinctions

It is essential to discuss briefly some of the ways in which we may distinguish between persons and non-persons simply because in research practice ethical issues arise from research with both persons and with animals. First, there are obvious differences between persons and machines although it has been proposed that some computers can think and have been referred to as artificial persons. Clearly computers do not share our human context which Wittgenstein called our forms of life. Computers do not share humour, companionship, pain and other regarding factors. According to Dreyfus (1981) our forms of life are part of our natural history and deeply embedded in our interpretative world. Three aspects of our human forms of life are important: human embodiment, possession of intrinsic interests and the capability to experience emotions in communication with others. A non-human organic being i.e. other animals, may share two out of three, whereas a machine does not share any. Furthermore, it is likely that the embryo may share at least one human embodiment of a rudimentary kind.

Rorty (1980) states that there is a widely held view supportive of a materialistic and functional approach in Artificial Intelligence that creatures can share the same mental states but differ radically in their internal makeup. If mental states are functional there is no appropriate reason why the same mental states cannot be realised in very different physical states i.e. in creatures of different species such as humans, dolphins and aliens. This allows for attribution of similar mental states to different biological and living organisms. However, in its extreme form of application, difficulties arise when applied to machines. Searle (1984) made a notable comment that if the functionalist view is applied to Artificial Intelligence then even a fountain pen with the right programme inputs would have a mind in the same sense as humans. According to Searle there is some emphasis upon the importance of having a biological body of some sort.

■ This sort of argument, at least justifies encouraging research by simulation through the use of computers.

Strawson (1959) remarks that animals are identified in causal rather than psychological terms. In other words, they do not have intentional states of mind and instinctually react. Nethertheless, Midgley (1983) claims that we know better than that, and we have no right to diminish the inner lives of the rest of creation. She defends the inner lives of non-language using animals by claiming that it may not be possible for the dog to say, 'it's time for tea', but it displays pleasure when its master turns up. From Midgley's point of view, this may be seen as a form of communication that indicates the pet dog does not react in only causal terms and its behaviour is meaningful. However, as well as Midgley giving other animals similar self-reflective features, she remarks that we may give creatures of our own kind preference in that it is a virtue to look after your own kind.

Whilst Midgley raises level of awareness in avoiding accepting a traditional model of 'the person', she argues that we may value our own kind first. However, these philosophical views are not sufficient for supporting the use of 'non-humans' or 'non-persons' in research practice. The ethical issues and concerns are still evident. If we 'value' ourselves and treat others like ourselves as 'persons', being 'persons' gives us the ability to be 'other regarding' to ourselves and to other sentient beings who share our life world. This means 'valuing' other animals. A moral value facilitates the principle of respect to other beings besides ourselves.

According to Kant, moral responsibility and free will are essential attributes of the person. Persons impose laws on themselves and are, therefore, worthy of respect. Sprague (1978) remarks that personal traits are important such as action, intending, perceiving, thinking and assigning responsibility. These are moral and psychological predicates. Sprague states that if we speak of versatile robots or chimpanzees who use American sign language (Washo) then it becomes difficult to withhold the title 'person' from a non-human entity. If this is the case, should animals be given rights of some sort? What will the consequences be in relation to animal experimentation? Is it the case that some animals have higher status than the human embryo?

The sciences and research

Our knowledge of human beings and of other beings in the world indicate similarities and differences. Empirical research takes its principles from the scientific domain. In chapter four, forms of knowledge were discussed. It is perhaps necessary to identify and synthesise basic ethical concerns in areas of knowledge and research.

Duffy (1985) remarks that nursing research utilises knowledge from the biological sciences (natural sciences) and social sciences. Nursing research may rely upon both the true experiment with the emphasis on the quantitative approach and the use of a qualitative approach which attempts to search for meaning, taking into account social and environmental factors. Nursing and Midwifery research also deals with people in diverse situations where respect for persons within research and professional practice must be central (cf chapter 5, 10, 11).

The positivist tradition lends itself to approaches which extend knowledge through generalising about the findings. The natural sciences are amenable to positivistic research because their subject matter can be broken down into parts and studied under laboratory conditions. Based upon the scientific or true experimental basis. Research is viewed as resting upon objective investigation, analysis from rational argument and observation of the facts. Cause and effect relationships are important. However, this form of research raises ethical issues and may be criticised if it is applied to persons and to some extent animal experimentation. Persons cannot be treated as objects or cells, organs or gases and therefore we cannot form generalisations easily. To measure or quantify or give meaningless numerical description is not only useless research but bad practice and negates scientific integrity. Misuse of quantitative methods, for example pre-scoring methods used in psychology for personality or intelligence tests, reduces personal experience to anonymity of mere numbers. The idea that a part of human nature can be explained by formalising intellectual understanding as complex facts and rules is highly implausible.

In areas of health care research, it may be said that although similarities exist between people, individual differences remain. Six people with the same diagnosis will think, feel and react differently depending on their individual biological, psychological and social experiences. It may not be sensible to 'extrapolate' from 'animal to man'. If differences occur between individual persons, obviously differences will exist between other species and ourselves.

Health care researchers and practitioners ought to be cautious in their choice and application of knowledge particularly within the behavioural sciences. A positivist approach in psychology may again serve as an example (cf chapter 4). However, it must be recognised that several psychological approaches are valuable within health care, notably social psychology that links closely to a social rather than a behavioural or positivist framework.

An extreme and controversial positivist perspective in psychology that uses 'animal experimentation' through the experimental research process, is neuroscience. Some psychologists themselves dispute that neuroscience is within a psychological framework. However, it is obvious that it is not within a social science framework. Neuroscience research includes the use of 'animal experimentation' for example, by humanely killing rats, in order to use brain tissue to trace chemicals across the neural pathways. If it is the case that animals are significantly different from the human, then surely only crude generalisations can be made in tracing the chemical journey through the rat's neural pathways. Animal experimentation is carried out, perhaps for its own sake, and constitutes 'trivial research'. Not only is this unethical but it raises the question of how far is it a contribution to knowledge for health or medical care? Should researchers endorse such research as contributing to 'acceptable research practice'?

There are differences between the subject matter of the natural sciences and those of the social sciences. These differences may show themselves through content and forms of explanation. However, good research practice allows for compatibility within the research process in that the ethical boundaries are common to both domains, specifically in medical and health care research.

Ethical boundaries: informed consent

Ethics in research is concerned with the rights of subjects or respondents. Many writers agree that informed consent is important particulary for autonomous 'humans'. The present author views informed consent as essential to research dealing with the person and central to health care research, particularly randomised clinical trials within the experimental domain. The key to moral dilemmas associated with clinical trials is consent and therefore deserves some discussion. (However, for detailed examination of the importance of informed-consent, readers are referred to chapter 7).

Faulder (1985) points out that thousands of patients are being entered into clinical trials without their knowledge and doctors justify their behaviour by saying that patients find it difficult to understand the scientific reasons for the study. For example, confidence will be undermined if a doctor has to confess that he or she does not know which treatment is best, hence the reason for a trial. Whilst this view mirrors paternalism in that the patient/respondent is passive and that the researcher/doctor knows best, it is clear that the absence of informed consent is of immediate concern. Person rights have been violated and may result in negative physical, psychological and emotional outcomes. Unfortunately, the patients are already stressed by illness.

Clinical trials may focus on those factors concerned with the improvement of health care. Scientific integrity also rests upon studies being well designed and likely to achieve answers. Morally, most health care workers will be faced with a dilemma between caring for the patient (the principle of benevolence) and caring for the majority (principle of utility). However, unless the autonomous person consents, the health care professional has no right to intervene at all (cf chapters 6 and 7).

There can be no justification for omitting to tell the subjects of their participation in research. However, the question arises what do we mean by informed consent? What would any of us want to know in order to make a decision regarding participation in research? The term informed consent is ambiguous and not readily defined or interpreted. Nevertheless it involves respect for autonomy of all persons. Informed consent ought to involve both implicit respect for persons whilst encouraging the researcher to evaluate his or her own motives regarding research interests. Consent involves sufficient information for informed choices to be made, recognising the disadvantaged situation of the patient by virtue of the illness, and diminution of personal autonomy. Where children are involved in research a further consideration would be a concern for the amount of information given to the child, especially when relatives have already given their consent.

Confidentiality concerns rights, privacy and respect for persons. However, the rules of confidentiality are not absolute simply because data has to be reported and requires public scrutiny. Nevertheless, 'anonymity' can be safeguarded.

Oakley (1990) remarks that the research process itself should not employ methods oppressive either to the researcher or the researched and should be oriented towards the production of knowledge. This is part of the formula for good practice. There has been a shift of value in both the natural and social sciences in that ethical issues are viewed as implicit within research practice. It is good research practitioners that produce the necessary quality in both understanding and explanation whilst extending the boundaries of knowledge.

Conclusion

In understanding what is meant by person status and its central focus within research practice, it seems that an analysis of personhood cannot be taken for granted, although to some extent it is guided by ordinary 'common-sense' use. In other words, in ordinary every day usage the term 'person' is co-extensive with human being. In common-sense every day use, we may not have a problem when it comes to questioning who should and who should not be counted as a person. In research practice, it may not be so straightforward. Generally speaking, humans are the only persons we recognise, therefore, there is little difficulty ascribing person status to humans. However, the embryo is certainly human and can be perceived as a potential person, although, it may be the case that some animals used in experimentation, may demand, on moral grounds, higher status than the embryo.

There are good reasons why person status should be discussed and understood further, particularly in relation to research practice. In person/non-person distinctions, adult subjects tend to indicate more abstract and rational construals. They are less contextually bound and may be influenced to some extent by their educational experience and professional training. It is obvious that professionals such as doctors, teachers and nurses are much more involved in research practice related to the caring environment and 'respect for persons' is central to their professional and research role. If the learning experience influences how we construe persons and non-persons, then it seems there is a strong argument for teaching ethical themes and research practice in higher education. Hargreaves (1980) asks the question, how do we modify 'commonsense' models and is understanding of a model necessary before modification occurs? Better understanding and modification occurs through education and generally raising levels of awareness. The outcome of developing a teaching scheme would have positive consequences for how we view others and ourselves, in the decision we make and in the action taken from those decisions. The more knowledge that is given and explored in thinking about the nature of persons, respect for persons and the ethical boundaries within research, the more direction is given to how we behave towards others.

The conception of the nature of persons has obviously more than one interpretation; for example, Dennett or Abelson's model, but the ascription of person status will command respect, rights and other moral and legal enactments. What may be of importance through educational initiatives, is the clarification of confusion and the encouragement of good research practice.

It is open to ourselves whether we give an individual person status or not. We can apply person status to non-humans, particularly if they are like ourselves in some way; according to Dreyfus sharing a form of life, or like Searle having a biological living body, or Kant, having an active human like mind. However, logic, language or observing behaviour cannot give the answer of who should or should not be given the title of 'person'. Respect comes with the status attached to the title of **personhood**. Abelson considers that persons are subjects of psychological and moral predicates. He also points out that the term is evaluative like the term 'good', therefore independent of biological classification. This makes it possible to ascribe person status to non-humans. Ideally, we ought to extend moral consideration to non-persons who share our world. It, therefore, follows that for developing confidence for the professional researcher, and raising ethical awareness for good research practice, the professional research curriculum ought to include debate of the issues of person/non-person distinctions. It expands the knowledge base, and our understanding of the more obscure ethical issues underpinning research practice in the natural sciences as well as in health care research generally.

References

Abelson R (1977). *Persons: A study in Philosophical Psychology*, Macmillan, London

Dennett D (1979). *Brainstorms,*Harvester Press, Sussex

Dreyfus R (1981). Micro worlds to Knowledge Representation: A1 at an Impasse, Haughland J ed, *Mind Design*, Bradford Books, Montgomery Vermont, pp 161-204

Duffy ME (1985). Designing Nursing Reserach: the qualitative quantitative debate, *J Adv Nurs*, **10**, 225-232

Faulder C (1985). *Whose Body is it,*Virgo Press, London.

Hargreaves D H (1980). Common-Sense Models of action, Chapman A and Jones D M ed, *Models of Man*, The British Psychological Society, Leicester, pp 215-225

Henry IC (1986). Conceptions of the nature of persons amongst children and adolescents, *Unpublished PhD*, Leeds University.

Midgley M (1983). *Animals and Why they matter: A journey around the species barrier*, Penguin, Harmondsworth.

Oakley A (1990). Who's afraid of the Randomised Controlled Trial? Some Dilemmas of Scientific Methed of Good Research Practice, Roberts? Helen ed, *Woman Health Accounts*, Routledge London p167-194.

Rorty R (1980). *Philosophy and the Mirror of Nature*, Basil Blackwell, Oxford

Ryle G (1949). *The Concept of Mind*, Penguin, Harmondsworth p61

Searle J (1984). *Reith Lectures: Mind, Brain and Science in the Listener*, BBC 15 November, p14-16

Sprague E (1978). *Metaphysical Thinking*, Oxford University Press, New York.

Strawson P F (1959). *Individuals*, Methuen, London.

Teichman J (1972). *Wittgenstein on Persons and Human beings in Understanding Wittgenstein*, Macmillan, London Royal Institute of Philosophy Lectures p133-148.

The British Psychological Society (1991). *Code of Conduct Ethical Principles and Guidelines* BPS 'Lecture', Warnock M (1985). A Question of Life, Blackwell, Oxford, p1-2.Warnock M (1985). *A Question of Life*, Blackwell, Oxford.

9 Reasonable care
Approaches to health care research
Christine Henry

Whilst the previous chapter explores in some depth ethical issues that may not be directly obvious, this chapter explores major principles and values inherent in good research practice. It attempts a synthesis of forms of knowledge and critically assesses approaches to health care research

Ethical issues can be examined in any environment and are not unique to health care research. Ethical principles, moral values and practice must be diversely but rigorously perceived within the parameters of what we mean by 'Community' (cf title of text). In order to formulate the framework in which to specifically discuss research in relation to Community Ethics, it may be appropriate to briefly identify and outline meanings of some general terms central to ethical practice and research.

Principles

Principles are guidelines for human conduct. They have a broad or universal application and may be viewed as essential to the way in which we behave towards each other. For example, how we would wish to be treated ourselves ought to influence how we treat others. From this one major principle arises, respect for persons. The term 'person' is value laden and, more specifically, is a moral term like 'good'. This has important implications for the ways in which we think about others like ourselves and, by consequence, the way we behave towards each other. If we deprive an individual in some way of their person status (in part, socially constructed) we deprived them of human rights, personal integrity, autonomy, the ability to make choices and individual responsibility. What happens for instance when the mentally handicapped person cannot make decisions for him/her self, or to the person who is so seriously ill that the nurse, practitioner, family and friends must take decisions on their behalf? Being another person's advocate is difficult. This is equally important for research practice within the health care setting. We all need to remember what happened in Nazi Germany when an ethnic group of people were treated as sub-human and denied person status. Many were used for experimental research and clearly classed as objects with little value.

Values

Values are much broader than principles and do not necessarily have to be moral. In Nazi Germany the officers who organised the exterminations in the concentration camps and likewise the soldiers who implemented the extermination process, shared values but not moral values. Moral values, on the other hand, are like maps that arise from our individual and social experiences. However, values have a subjective and personal interpretation and can violate or support **principles** and in turn, professional or research practice.

Ethics

Ethics assess the ways in which we behave and the quality of the moral values we have (EVA 1992). Ethics, nevertheless, give us a tool for enquiring into our behaviour and whilst not giving right or wrong answers, may give moral justifications for actions and choices. The use of ethical theories may help to resolve conflict between alternative actions. Nevertheless, applying one ethical theory to a specific health care situation may not be sufficient in itself. In 'Common-sense' terms and through everyday language, morals and ethics are used to mean the same thing. Morals concern human conduct and values whereas ethics is the study of both conduct and values. There are many ethical issues that share common ground within the community and the professional and research field.

Professional Ethics

Professional Ethics specifically may be said to derive from ethics in that it considers the way in which professionals practise. Professional ethics encourages guidelines for professional conduct in care and research practice. Furthermore, professional ethics applied to research practice deals with ethical concerns related to the power, role and position of professionals or researchers for example, gaining informed consent and the consequences of this (cf chapter 7). Priority in research practice must always be respect for persons, encouraging personal autonomy and the right to refuse to participate in the research project. According to Broad (1991) focus on the scholarship of discovery makes the researcher accountable to the community. This is further emphasised if the Professional is the researcher. Wilcox and Ebbs (1992) remark that knowledge is a 'communal affair' which does not just involve personal integrity in the ward or laboratory or that of being a mentor or role model for students. The researcher is an integral member of the profession, the organisation and the wider social community. Clearly professional integrity and accountability are concerned with the processes and practices of research. Research projects in Nursing and Health, by their very nature, have a community focus, especially if they involve improving care. Professional Ethics encourages multidisciplinary involvement with other social and health care professionals in the nature and process of discovery and scholarship. Some outcomes from research and its managed process may identify standards and help to support the need for developing a Code of Conduct for Research Practice. There is no such thing as 'values free' research since research presupposes a set of values. Deceptive research can be challenged on two accounts: the integrity of the research project itself and the dignity of those deceived Bok, (1983).

The question arises how can we serve the public in the way they need, without conflict between personal ethics and values and the ethics of our professional or researcher's role?

It is important to look at some specific issues that surround two disparate forms or explanations used in health care research. A brief overview of the concept of care and person leads into a discussion of a research approach that enhances understanding rather than prediction and generalisation and in turn raises levels of ethical awareness in research practice.

Often we demand natural explanations of disease and give an account of insanity by reducing statements and behaviour produced by the person to the consequences of pathology (cause and effect explanations). However, in matters of normal everyday life we demand accounts of statements and behaviour in terms of reasons and values, for example, we do not see crime and sin as pathological or on a par with those produced by certain diseases. The person is free and responsible for his/her actions and behaviour. This relates closely to the idea that a person is seen as an active agent and involves treating the person as autonomous and author of his/her own actions as far as is possible. (Although it is worth noting that the term 'autonomy' is an ideal concept).

Respect for persons is the main focus for the caring professions and the emphasis may surround not only reasons and moral value but also how the person interprets his/her situation. Cause and effect explanations relate to the natural world whereas reasons relate to the human mind and persons interacting with each other in the world. There is an appropriate and proper place within the research field for 'cause and effect' explanations. However, values are not facts and reasons are not causes. Downie and Telfer (1980) remark that on first sight medicine is based on the natural sciences, whereas social work is based on the social sciences. Various health professions will use knowledge from both domains. This can cause some conflict for the health professional because of the nature of the two diverse forms of knowledge (cf chapter 4). Downie and Telfer correctly point out that natural science explanations of the world are based upon the concept of a thing and this in turn involves explanations based upon causal relationships. An example could be the identification of a particular microbe that may cause disease. The microbe in this sense is conceptualised as a thing, a biological organism. However, within the social sciences there is uncertainty regarding causal relationships and lawlike generalisations that may be used in order to understand persons. Persons cannot be treated as things in a simple cause and effect relationship: persons are not things. It has already been mentioned in the previous chapter how other species through experimentation can be treated as objects with no value or status (cf chapter 8).

The central focus for the applied social sciences and humanities utilised in health and social care practice must be the 'Person'. A related concept is the value concept of care, of essential importance to professional practice and to subsequent research practice by the professional. One way of emphasising the difference between conceptualisations in medical practice and nursing practice, respectively, can be shown as in Table 9.1.

Table 9.1 'Care and Cure'

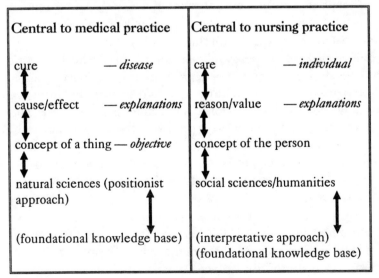

In medical practice, the concept of care is important but not central to the model. However, the concept of care is central to nursing practice having moral and social value.

The concept of care is difficult to define but it is important to remember that the moral/value elements link closely with respect for persons and the meaning we give to a concept may depend upon how we use it (Henry 1986). The concept of care is very similar to how we use the term 'human' in that the term has a semi-normative and descriptive element to it, for example, the descriptive element refers to being human and a member of a biological species, whereas the semi-normative element is the value we place on having human/person features. The concept of care could have a descriptive element in the technical sense, for example, in caring for your teeth, describing brushing and physical care and treatment, and a semi-normative element in value placed upon the caring for you as a person for yourself, and by the professional, i.e. dentist.

The term 'care' is linked to the term 'person' through the evaluative features, and in meaning and use related to respect for persons. Whilst it is not easy to define, it functions within our Common-Sense world of everyday experience. The concept of care from our interpretative world, can be a junior partner/relative/cousin to the concept of a person.

Medical education still clings firmly to the natural sciences whilst there is an uneasy relationship within the health carer's curriculum between the biological and social science. This is, in part, due to the nature and diversity of the forms of knowledge. Biological science for instance is still essential and remains central to medicine if practice is based upon diagnosis. However, in understanding the person as a whole, the social sciences and the humanities are equally important to the practice of health care, generally for the doctor, and specifically for the nurse.

In order to expand our body of knowledge and increase our understanding research must be seen as essential for the caring professions. A phenomenological perspective which offers an alternative to traditional experimental research within the natural sciences, fits more appropriately with health care and the concept of the person. The concepts of care and person are not easily defined, both are evaluative and rest upon meaning and interpretation. If this is the case, both concepts are more appropriately foundational to the social sciences and humanities. This supports a phenomenological perspective.

Social science enquiry is not the same as natural or physical science forms of enquiry although the research processes may similarly avoid subjective bias, and seek validity. The social sciences have become less positivistic and much more interpretative.

Before explaining and identifying the main features of the phenomenological approach in health care research, it would be useful to outline the main features of the traditional positivist approach originating within the natural science domains in order to clarify related elements of a traditional research practice, often used in both medical and some health care research .

Positivism

An approach founded upon the *Positivist* tradition can easily be viewed as reducing people to things and cannot provide a satisfactory understanding of human life alone. It cannot give a clear understanding of a person's experience through illness and health. Positivism aims to be scientific and data is collected in order to test an hypothesis. This involves observation and controlled experiments in order to be descriptive, objective and to make predictions and generalisations. For the positivists, causal explanations are important. It is from this approach that medical science will utilise controlled experimental methods, e.g. clinical trials. In the medical field and some health care domains this approach can generate some useful information particularly in terms of physiological changes, for example in wound-healing procedures with new forms of treatment. The positivist view can reflect a reductionist and materialist perspective and the individual is seen only in physiological terms (Henry and Pashley 1990). (An important point at this stage is to be reminded that the term 'person' is a term and not open to biological classification. In other words, not a descriptive category but a 'value term'). It is not a natural concept that can be descriptive and classified like the term *Homo-Sapien* (being a member of a biological species). It is also essential to remember that the concern in most areas of health care research involves consideration of the person as a whole, especially if the concept of care is central to professional practice.

What is missing from an experimental approach is the unobservable phenomena that will influence behaviour, such as motives, feelings, thoughts, intentions, decisions, personality and experience and these are all person features. These person features whilst viewed as more subjective, are open to meaning and interpretation rather than cause and effect explanations.

It seems that there is a crude division between the positivist experimental approach on one side and the highly humanisitic rational and sometimes subjective approach on the other. However, if we advocate a research approach in health care concerned with the person viewed as more than the sum of his/her parts, there is some requirement to compromise between the two disparate approaches. A sensible foundation would be a phenomenological perspective.

A Phenomenological Perspective

A phenomenological perspective treats 'common sense' knowledge as the principle topic for study and therefore relates closely to matters of normal conduct based upon understanding. The person is seen as active and experience is considered important, with emphasis upon meaning and interpretation. Husserl (1858-1938) was the founder of the phenomenological approach and his central concept is that of everyday experience. Bolton (1979) remarks that in taking a phenomenological approach, the objective is subjectively constituted, *viz.* we make interpretations on the world and ourselves.

Observing that there are similarities between people in health and illness, as well as individual differences in their perceptions and constructs, the phenomenological approach, whilst not attempting to establish facts about human nature, will utilise objective methods of research applied to the subject matter, be it experience or behaviour. This research approach has a set of procedures to overcome conjecture and 'commonsense' intuition. Most contemporary researchers advocate the use of objective forms of enquiry, even if the researcher studies intentions and subjective experiences. What ought to be avoided is the application of quantatification and predictability upon highly evaluative and qualitative person features. The subject matter, i.e. person, is more complex than that of physics or biology. (The behaviour of things such as atoms or microbes is more predictable). The traditional physical sciences stemming from the positivist view insists that a variable is something that can be measured as part of the system being studied. For example when a chemical substance does not interact with another substance, prediction is easy. However, it is not as simple with person features. It may be viewed that psychological variables are difficult to identify and are not objects in the structural sense. Furthermore, they cannot easily be isolated from their complex interactive role in the changing active person.

In the health care system, there is difficulty in explaining the whole person in terms of his/her parts. Whilst it is obvious that the physical world along with its attendant pathological diseases will affect or influence how a person feels, behaves and acts, it is not the same thing as experimental researchers giving explanations of higher order features of the person through causal relationships. The consequences of measuring person features like intelligence results in ethical concerns for research practice. It not only can result in treating 'persons' as objects but also in poor research outcomes that may be implemented to the detriment of care, for example, accepting without question, and without identifying the many other variables such as prescribing vitamins to improve a child's level of intelligence. Whilst it is obvious that malnutrition or a consistently poor diet will influence ability, it is not a written absolute truth or certainty that taking vitamins will increase a child's intelligence.

Methods

Most researchers are now less dogmatic about methods used to collect data. However, all methods of collecting data involving persons and their interactions are basically problematical. Valentine (1982) remarks that no method guarantees certainty.

Measurement has been seen as central to the experimental scientific domain but it is perhaps clear that measurements of psychological phenomena is difficult. According to Howarth (1981) measurement need not be quality to be useful, for example broad judgements of 'greater than or less than'. These can be seen to quantify and describe in a primitive form responses to attitude scales such as degrees of liking or disliking. The researcher who focuses upon the person's meaning or interpretation in a health care situation may use this primitive form of measurement to summarise identifiable responses within a particular setting or context and at a given time. However, what ought to be avoided are measurements of individual differences such as intelligence or personality traits, especially if the person is ill and cognitive functioning and personality may be influenced by his/her illness. Howarth remarks that measurement is neutral and meaning is given to the data by the researcher.

Duffy (1985) remarks that there are two disparate approaches in research practice: on the one hand research that relates to the true experiment which is within the positivist tradition and on the other research that avoids measurement and predictability and which has a phenomenological framework. An extreme positivist approach will seek to verify facts emphasising causal relationships and give little regard to subjective states of persons. The goal is to establish general laws common to the phenomenon regardless of the setting. The methods seek to reduce and isolate the variables. It is therefore important not to use this traditional approach in some research if the focus is upon meaning and interpretation. Mismatch of methods to the research focus result in 'bad research'.

The main focus of the phenomenological perspective is understanding human behaviour from the agent's perspective and the person's experience of everyday life events (Field and Morse 1985). Data is analysed through more subjective interpretations and is not open to statistical analysis in the objective sense. However, what is helpful is using more than one method for collecting data. The researcher may concentrate upon the generation of theory through information obtained within the 'natural setting', *viz*. the ward. Furthermore, the researcher will have to recognise that the complex interacting social variables will influence human behaviour, for example, the local hospital environment. In carrying out research the researcher seeks to understand the facts by getting inside the natural setting and becoming involved in the social context, whether it be the hospital ward or the community setting. Methods such as participant observation, non- participant observation, open ended interview techniques, case study methods and action research approaches are all useful in taking a phenomenological approach in research.

Winch (1958) states that we may understand a piece of behaviour only when there is some possibility of choice and this emphasises that the person is active and free rather than reactive and determined. Winch goes on to remark that human behaviour is rule governed and it is impossible to make scientific laws about behaviour of an agent whose actions themselves determine the rules under which he/she acts. Perhaps the important point to make is that different research approaches should or ought to be used to match what is being studied. If research in the health care field focuses upon meaning and interpretation from the agent's perspective, which obviously involves 'person' constructs, then this approach for research practice may have more to offer than traditional experimental approach.

References

Bolton N, 1970. *Philosophical problems in Psychology,* Methuen.

Bok D 1990. *Universities and the Future of America- Durham NC,* Duke University Press

Broad W J 1991. Cold Fusion Claim is Faulted on Ethics as well as Science, *New York Times.*

Downie R S and Telfer E 1980. *Caring and Curing,* Methuen; London

Duffy M 1985. Designing Nursing Research the qualitative-quantitative debate, *J Adv Nurs,* **10**, 225-232.

Field P A and Morse J M 1985. *Nursing research: The application of Qualitative Research,* Croom Helm, London.

Henry I C 1986. Conceptions of the nature of Persons, *Unpublished PhD,* Leeds University.

Henry I C and Pashley G 1990. *Health Care Research,* Quay Publishing, Lancaster.

Howarth C I 1981. The nature of psychological knowledge, Howarth C I and Gillham W E eds, *The Structure of Psychology,* George Allen Unwin London, pp 3-16

Valentine E 1982. *Conceptual Issues in Psychology,* George Allen Unwin: London.

Winch P 1958. *The Idea of a Social Science,* Routledge and Kegan Paul: London.

Wilcox J R and Ebbs S L 1992. *The leadership Compass:- Values and Ethics in Higher Education,* The George Washington University, Washington DC

10 Nursing research
Time for an educational strategy
June Davison

This chapter explores current approaches to nursing education and addresses issues on how to improve professional research practice by preparing the potential professional practitioner/researcher. It debates, in some depth, the curriculum and further addresses the role and accountability of the professional nurse educators.

The aims of this chapter are to explore the concept of research competency within the nursing profession, to question the perceived lack of strategic planning for research methodology training and to address the issue of liaison between the health care environment and educational institutions.

The need to strengthen links between researchers, nurse educationalists and nurse practitioners is emphasised with a view to improving communications, narrowing the theory/practice gap and realistically identifying needs in terms of research methodology training and professional development.

The teaching of research to pre-registration student nurses is also discussed and highlights the need to be innovative in the teaching methods used and not to view the concept of research as a 'stand alone' topic, but as an integrated component of the theory and practice of nursing. The ethical issues are implicit with value placed upon educating the professional nurse to 'care' in both practice and research.

Introduction

Most philosophies of care evolve from a fundamental premise which is to meet the needs of individuals who require some form of action in relation to either promotion of health, or minimising the effects of ill health. The aims of the educational process for nursing seek to facilitate the development of a nurse/practitioner who, working as a member of the multidisciplinary team, has the skills to identify the problems of clients and plan and implement care appropriate to individual needs. In order to achieve the optimum care in terms of quality, the nurse needs to have the knowledge and skills to discriminate between what is good and what is bad in nursing practice and research. The promotion of knowledge and the development of skills should be founded on the basis of relevant and accepted research findings, and the learning experiences within educational programmes should be facilitated by well prepared teaching staff, who themselves have the requisite knowledge and skills in professional and research practice.

Historically, research into health care was not seen as the prime responsibility of nurses, but in recent years, there has been a move towards a growing 'body of knowledge', researched and developed by an increasing number of nurses committed to seeking ways of improving health care both directly and indirectly. Unfortunately, as the number of nurses involved in research increased, so did the diversity of the nature and quality of some research programmes. 'Research' has become a vogue word and whilst it should be associated with progressive thinking, many people have realised the need to pay 'lip service' to it as a means of achieving personal development. This is an ethical issue and is an integral part of being a 'professional'.

Research competency

Many of the post-registration courses in nursing and other health related subjects do have a varying degree of input related to research methodology. However, the levels of research competency achieved must be questionable and very dependent upon a wide range of factors including facilities, time and the availability of expert teaching and supervision. If an educational strategy for nursing research exists within the profession, then it is time to explore the motives underlying this strategy in order to minimise the diverse nature and sometimes questionable quality of some of the work.

Quality enhancement as an ethical foundation

It is a current trend within professional and educational circles to favour the use of the word 'educate' rather than 'train'. However, on examining the Oxford dictionary definition of the two words, it would appear, in literal terms, that the words 'train' and 'educate' are synonymous. To train is 'to bring to desired state or standard of efficiency by instruction and practice' and to educate is 'to train intellectually and morally'. The differences between training and education could be, and indeed are, argued on a much more sophisticated, complex and philosophical level, but for the purpose of this chapter the word 'training' should be accepted in its broadest sense. The term 'training' implies moral features and perhaps refers to 'practising what we preach'. We probably make the mistake of separating out both terms 'training' and 'education'.

There does not appear to be a recognised standard to education/training in research methodology and much reliance is made upon the validating bodies of courses offering research options. Training may range from a full time degree course exploring the many facets of research methods, to the 'lip service' paid in many other health related lower level courses.

Is there an accepted model of competence in research training and do all sections of the health care work force require the same level of competence? Different components of the work force require different levels of ability in terms of carrying out and implementing a programme of relevant research. Not everyone needs skills to identify research problems and make decisions regarding methods, implementation and possible policy statements.

In the health service, training in research methods has resource implications at all levels, e.g. at the most simplistic level, course fees, release from work and lecture fees. Thought should be given to how these resources are most effectively utilised, as expensive training research methods is not the only way forward. Research awareness and skills to implement research findings are just as important to the improvement of health care, and it would be of value to assess the current status of research not only in nursing but in the health service as a whole. Health care is multidisciplinary and members of the work force should be exploring not only their own fields of research, but also those of other disciplines aiming to minimise duplication of work and promote more effective utilisation of resources. Precisely because health care is 'multidisciplinary' highlights the ethical concerns involved in 'watered down' duplicity which results in 'poor research'.

The professions have a lot of gain from research collaboration, not least, an increased level of research competency. Research competency is essential for 'professional recognition'. It will ensure improvement in quality of care.

Exploring the National Health Service Research and Development Strategy

Research for Health (DHSS, 1991). states that the objective of the NHS Research and Development Strategy is:

To ensure that the content and the delivery of care in the NHS is based on high quality research relevant to improving the health of the nation and that its success is partially dependent upon a well trained work force to carry out the programme. A corollary of this is the provision of appropriate training in research methods and it is suggested that such issues are addressed by medical schools and other institutions with responsibilities for training/education.

Institutions with responsibilities for training/education in health care include universities with or without medical schools, further education colleges and colleges of nursing, midwifery and health studies (though many of the latter are now integral parts of higher education).

The health care work force is multidisciplinary and training occurs at a variety of levels ranging from health care assistants working towards National Vocational Training Schemes, receiving a role-based competency type of training, who should be encouraged to develop research awareness in order to deliver relevant care. This section of the Health Service work force are in direct contact with clients and should be aware of the rationale behind the care they are giving. Research findings related to the safe lifting and handling of patients (Bell, 1984), the appropriate methods of mouth care (Crosby, 1989) and current practices in pressure area care David *et al*, 1983) are examples that could be used in the education/training programmes of ward-based health care assistants.

In the interest of quality, there is a need to keep all sections of the work force updated in current health care practices and in particular the people who have direct client contact. These are not only the doctors, nurses physiotherapists and other professionals, but also the porters and other ancillary staff. The health service should recognise the need to fund regular update sessions for this section of the work force as these are the people who need to know about maintaining a safe environment by, for example, the safe disposal of dangerous waste material (Simmons, 1983) and by encouraging safe practices in the cleaning of the health care environment (World Health Organisation, 1978). Much research has been funded in this area and has influenced policies on maintaining a safe environment (Department of Health, 1990); it is illogical to think that the very people who are employed to maintain a safe environment are not made aware of the reasons for their working practices. It could be argued that unit policies exist and are accessible to everyone, but how many people really understand the implications of their actions?

An 'Update Day', maybe on an annual basis, for porters and ancillary staff could provide a venue for discussion of work practices and why they need to perform accurately in terms of safety procedures. Ownership of quality care and standards does not belong exclusively to the professionals and management. However, it may be that the professionals are held accountable (cf chapters 2 and 3).

Even though the support and ancillary section of the health care work force are not recognised as having a need for training in research methods, they should, nevertheless, have the opportunity to develop a working knowledge of the rationale underlying their work practices.

Education/Training in research methods for post-registration nurses

Though the health care work force is multidisciplinary in nature and offers care in a variety of institutional and non-institutional settings, nurses form a very large proportion of this work force. Many of these are directly or indirectly involved with health care research with involvement ranging from assisting in data collection for other researchers' projects, to conducting research programmes of their own.

Many nurses in the past have been employed under the title of 'research nurse' mostly to assist (particularly in medical research) the main researcher with data collection, clinics or other client matters. The nurses in question would not have research methods training, but would have learnt the appropriate task-oriented skills of their particular roles whilst in post. Quite often and quite rightly, these research nurses would have no input into the resulting research report, but would be acknowledged with thanks at publication. How ethical is this?

Such research nursing posts are still advertised today (Nursing Times, 1992) and the nurses applying for them should recognise and take the opportunity to find ways of educating in order to increase their own skills in research methods, as well as opening up avenues into the realms of the systematic exploration of health care. The true role of a 'research nurse' encompasses far more than the collection of data and, if this is all that is offered in a research nursing post, then consideration should be given to changing the title of the post to something more appropriate.

There are many well motivated and innovative nurses who do question the way in which care is organised and implemented and, given the opportunity, skills and resources would systematically explore the rationale behind the care they are giving. They could also be instrumental in changing practice if the changes could be justified and supported by the findings of a credible and skilful study. Unfortunately, owing to the pressure of working in circumstances where lack of resources means less time for study leave and professional development, nurses can become complacent about innovation and 'increasing the body of nursing knowledge'.

There is also the scenario, where nurses are released, one day a week, to attend courses leading to post-registration qualifications and it is possible that some of these courses will include a research element. A requirement of the course may be to complete a 'small scale research project'. Quite often, because of the conflicting demands of trying to maintain a full time commitment to a job and trying to come to terms with the complexities of research methods on a one day a week basis, trying to complete a research project may create so much anxiety and stress that the nurse ends up feeling exhausted, confused and reluctant to attempt to research practice again.

It is also important how these courses are taught. The teachers must not only be credible in research practice themselves, but must find ways of motivating and encouraging research mindedness.

Many return to their particular areas of practice with a certificate or diploma and a research project that will probably never be read by anyone else and any attempts at implementation of the findings can prove futile, particularly in areas where there are long established traditions of customs and practice.

This is not the ideal way of educating nurses in research methods. Researchers need time to think, to read and develop the right research approach to their area of enquiry and explore the feasibility of implementing any relevant findings in their area of practice; otherwise, the whole process becomes a paper exercise in the interest of 'research methods' as a means to personal development. Personal development is not always synonymous with professional development, hence the emphasis of an integrated curriculum for research with professional and ethical themes.

There is no doubt that there are many talented, experienced and skilful nurse researchers working to increase the body of nursing knowledge and there is also no doubt that there are many academic nurses who are not in direct contact with clients. The gap between nursing theory and nursing practice is a constant source of discussion (Van Maanen, 1979) and though clinically based nurses and nurse educationalists strive to narrow this gap, it is still very much evidence.

There are many reasons as to why the gap is perpetuated, one of these being that the more academically successful the nurse/researcher becomes, the more likely this individual is to leave the health care arena to enter full time educational pursuits and join the realms of academic excellence. Because of the commitment necessary to such work, it is understandable that the nurse/researcher develops a different set of skills to replace declining and possibly outdated clinical skills. As nurses develop their academic expertise, individual potential, in terms of research awareness and research methods skills, must increase. It is through identifying the 'shared values' through both practice and research that the diversity may be overcome.

The disadvantages of nurse/researchers moving away from the health care environment, include decreasing working knowledge of the health care practices that may be improved by systematic enquiry. If there is to be a co-ordinated approach to identifying research problems, researcher must maintain an awareness of, and be in touch with current health care and how it is implemented, not just through reading but through the development of meaningful links with the health care environment. Once again, this raises an ethical concern.

Decreasing the theory–practice gap

Academic research staff need to know the problems require researching and have the skills to design research projects and select and use the appropriate methodology. Nurse practitioners need to have an increased awareness of and the ability to identify researchable problems; they also require the skills to analyse, evaluate and implement relevant findings. Nurse educationalists need to have the skills to facilitate learning in terms of health care research, its relevance and its implementation.

Strong and effective links between the health care environment, colleges of nursing and higher education institutions are essential in order to decrease the theory–practice gap. Nurse practitioners, nurse educationalists and academic staff have much to learn from one another. A particular strength on the side of the nurse practitioners and the nurse educationalists is the existence of well established liaison links with health care environments and a strength of the academic staff lies in their well established expertise in research methods.

Liaison models

The development of an education/service liaison model could help narrow the theory–gap and enhance the quality of communication at both an interpersonal and departmental level. Some colleges of nursing and health studies already have well established clinical liaison standards and when all such colleges have become totally integrated within institutes of higher education, there will be an even greater need to develop and strengthen such liaison standards, not only to promote research awareness and training, but to ensure that academic staff, researchers, nurse educationalists and nurse practitioners maintain a dialogue regarding the provision of high quality health care. It is also important to maintain liaison regarding the updating and professional development needs of those working in the health care environment and those working in educational institutions.

Higher education liaison links

There is a current initiative underway to integrate all colleges of nursing and midwifery into institutes of higher education. The dangers of such a move include a possible weakening of links with practitioners. Thus, it is essential to promote a liaison model from the very outset of the integration. Consideration must be given to the ways in which communication channels will interface with already established networks within higher education.

Figure 1 shows how the Newcastle liaison model could be extended to institutes of higher education and function in relation to both pre-registration and post-registration health care courses including nursing and midwifery.

It is important to have an effective liaison model, not only to monitor the health care environment and the support of students on placements, but also to assess the needs of the practitioners in terms of research methods training and attempt

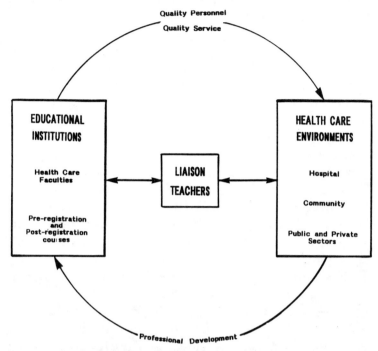

Figure 10.1 Education-service liaison model

to facilitate strategies aimed at increasing research awareness and promoting the implementation of findings.

This gives the added dimension of research to the liaison role and one which may create initial difficulties if the teachers do not possess the right level of academic skills. Many nurse teachers do have academic skills, acquired through graduate courses. However, some may need the extra support that should be available from research staff within the institutes of higher education. This linking of practitioners, nurse teachers and research staff could lead to a co-ordinated approach to research methodology training and professional development.

It could be argued that the opportunity for professional development for nurse practitioners is limited owing to lack of resources and pressure of work, however, there are many ways in which knowledge can be updated and skills acquired. It is not always necessary to attend educational institutions to gain further qualifications. There are many excellent alternatives such as open and distance learning packages supported by tutorial systems. Unfortunately, some of these are quite expensive which limits access unless funds can be negotiated through various channels. A co-ordinated approach in planning to meet the continuing education needs of nurses has been an on-going objective for the English National Board for Nursing, Midwifery and Health Visiting (ENB) for some time.

The launch of the ENB *Framework for Continuing Professional Education and Higher Awards* (ENB, 1992a) was in response to the ENB's Training Needs Analysis Project and could provide many nurse practitioners with the necessary flexible approach to professional development. There is tremendous potential here for many nurse practitioners to capitalise, in a structured way, on this initiative as one of the aims is to give recognition for what has already been accomplished by an individual and prevent repetitious learning. However, it is still in its very early stages and how it is to be implemented has not yet, in many areas, been clarified. A way forward could be through use of the education/service liaison links, the clinical liaison teachers acting as advisers and enablers, seeking help from researchers and other educationalists to work with nurse practitioners in identifying unit strategies for preparing and submitting professional portfolios.

An aim of the framework is to:

Ensure that practitioners maintain and develop their skills in providing high quality care and increase their contribution to ensuring that health care providers achieve their quality targets relating to meeting the changing health care needs of the population.

Changing health care needs of the population mean changing health care practices and this involves the exploration and evaluation of current health care practices through research. High quality care should be based on a well developed body of relevant knowledge and delivered by practitioners with the skills to not utilise that knowledge base but also to constantly question it and, where relevant, change it.

The teaching of research methods to post-registration nurse practitioners should be approached with a sensitivity to individual need and, as already mentioned, the level of competency required will depend on the context in which the practitioner will be expected to use research.

The development and implementation of Project 2000 curricula has provided the opportunity to develop a strategy for educating student nurses in terms of research methods, hopefully providing them with a sound basis from which they can progress as qualified practitioners.

Teaching research to nursing students

The ENB and the Council for National Academic Awards provided guidelines for the development of pre-registration nursing courses (ENB, 1992b) and these guidelines suggest that:

> *The research basis of knowledge should inform the teaching of a course right from the beginning and students will attain a deeper understanding of research results as the course progresses. By the end of the course, the diplomat is seen as the analytical consumer of research results but not yet capable of starting to do research.*

The same guidelines suggest the need for collaborative research links between staff in colleges of nursing and midwifery and institutions of higher education. It is disappointing that the importance of links with nurse practitioners is not fully emphasised in this document.

Descriptions of the Major Categories in the Cognitive Domain (BLOOM 1956)

---

1. Knowledge. Knowledge is defined as the remembering of previously learned material. This may involve the recall of a wide range of material, from specific facts to complete theories, but all that is required is the bringing to mind of the appropriate information. Knowledge represents the lowest level of learning outcomes in the cognitive domain.

---

2. Comprehension. Comprehension is defined as the ability to grasp the meaning of material. This may be shown by translating material from one form to another (words to numbers), by interpreting material) explaining or summarizing), and by estimating future trends (predicting consequences or effects). These learning outcomes go one step beyond the simple remembering of material, and represent the lowest level of understanding.

---

3. Application. Application refers to the ability to use learned material in new and concrete situations. This may include the application of such things as rules, methods, concepts, principles, laws and theories. Learning outcomes in this area require a higher level of understanding than those under comprehension.

---

4. Analysis. Analysis refers to the ability to break down material into its component parts so that its organizational structure may be understood. This may include the identification of the parts, analysis of the relationships between parts, and recognition of the organizational principles involved. Learning outcomes here represent a higher intellectual level than comprehension and application because they require an understanding of both the content and the structural form of the material.

---

5. Synthesis. Synthesis refers to the ability to put parts together to form a new whole. This may involve the production of a unique communication (theme or speech), a plan of operations (research proposal), or a set of abstract relations (scheme for classifying information). Learning outcomes in this area stress creative behaviours, with major emphasis on the formulation of new patterns or structures.

---

6. Evaluation. Evaluation is concerned with the ability to judge the value of material (statement, novel, poem, research report) for a given purpose. The judgements are to be based on definite criteria. These may be internal criteria (organisation) or external criteria (relevance to the purpose) and the student may determine the criteria or be given them. Learning outcomes in this area are highest in the cognitive hierarchy because they contain elements of all of the other categories, plus conscious value judgements based on clearly defined criteria.

Fig. 10.2 Description of the major categories in the cognitive domain (Bloom, 1956)

Nursing research cannot be taught as a 'stand alone' topic within the curriculum, it must be taught in such a way that it becomes alive and dynamic and can be easily applied to the practice of nursing. This is easier said than done owing to the rigid way in which some curricula are written and interpreted. It would seem that many validating bodies like to see the research component of pre-registration courses articulated in a structured and easy-to-follow format. There is no doubt that there is a need to identify the level of competence being aimed for within the course outcomes and that this is addressed through the design of the assessment strategy. However, teachers and lecturers should be allowed to be innovative in the ways in which the research outcomes are met.

With an assessment strategy based on, for example, the taxonomy of Bloom (1956), the student passes through stages of cognitive achievement ranging from knowledge and comprehension, to synthesis and evaluation; there is an identified structure within which the student can be placed according to the stage of an individual achievement (see Figure 2). Some students may achieve one stage more rapidly than another, it would be unrealistic to assume that all students progress through the same developmental process together. This highlights the importance of having flexibility within an educational programme to allow students to progress at their own pace. Research is a good example of a topic that could be taught in this individualistic way.

The way that student nurses are introduced to research is very important owing to the complex nature of the topic. There have been many approaches to teaching the theory and practice of research. However, there are certain questions that should be addressed before the design stage of any research teaching programme.

- What do student nurses need to know about research?
- What methods should be used to teach research to student nurses and who should do the teaching?
- How should the level of student achievement be assessed?

- What should the level of student achievement be?

- What should be the content of the research curriculum? Should ethical issues be clearly identified specifically to research practice?

What do student nurses need to know about research?

Student nurses need to know the meaning and purpose of research and explore the ways in which nursing theories and research interface with nursing practice and the professionalisation of nursing.

There is a need to explore what is meant by the 'research process', the ethical practice of research and how this is translated into research methods. Various research methods should be explored, such as qualitative, quantitative and ethnographic as well as a general introduction to some of the less well used methods such as the idiographic and hermeneutic approach as described by Thomas (1984).

Students need to develop a working knowledge of the general structures used in the writing of research reports and ultimately have the skills to evaluate and implement relevant findings.

There is an urgent need for students to perceive research as an integral component of nursing studies and to feel comfortable in terms of including recent research findings to support their rationale when planning and implementing care. They should feel equally comfortable in criticising research in terms of its quality and relevance.

What methods should be used to teach research to student nurses and who should do the teaching?

Methods of teaching nursing research vary considerably between individuals and between institutes teaching nursing, but the current trend towards a 'student centred approach' has opened up new and often innovative doors to the teaching and learning process.

The concept of well supported self-directed learning is one that allows students to develop cognitive skills and grow in academic confidence. Unfortunately, this method can be abused and act as an opt-out situation for some teachers unless there is a well defined self-directed study strategy agreed between student and teacher.

A self-directed student requires a clear indication of what must be achieved and have access to the resources necessary to achieve the identified outcomes. Thus, well referenced study guides and appropriate set texts in the libraries are important aids to the student. It is essential to have effective liaison with librarians so that they can co-operate as far as possible in identifying and making available the necessary reading materials. The student mentors working in the health care environment should be aware of what the student is trying to achieve and should also have access to the same resources. The liaison teacher can act as a supportive link in this process, attempting to link theory and practice.

Seminars and tutorials can help provide peer group and teacher support in the facilitation of learning about research and adequate supervision and feedback are important to the progression of students when they are exploring complicated concepts. Unfortunately, colleges of nursing do not always have the research expertise to teach to the required diploma level and must, therefore, acknowledge these deficits and, where possible, 'contract in' the necessary lecturers from higher education institutions to deal with this until nurse teachers have reached degree level themselves through professional development programmes.

This deficit in research expertise, is not always acknowledged and can cause problems in the quality of research teaching and student supervision provided. Traditionally, it is common for nurse teachers to become possessive with their students and try to meet all academic needs as an individual. This can be problematical and nurse teachers should be encouraged to use the expertise available and work side by side with others to achieve the best possible learning experience for the student.

The self-directed method of learning can be well adapted to meeting the research needs of the student, particularly in exploring the principles underlying research methodology.

It is unrealistic to suppose that student nurses are encouraged to actually carry out and write up a piece of research, considering the time it would take and the resources it would require. Quality research requires the correct level of supervision and guidance through the many pathways involved, such as the research and ethical committees, the consideration of theoretical frameworks and the project design. If individuals are to produce a worthwhile project, worthy of consideration for changing policy or practice, it should not be done during a pre-registration course, where coping with the sheer numbers of students could be counter-productive in terms of goals. Pre-registration students have many competencies in order to provide high quality patient care, competency in research methodology should be a natural progression in post-registration development.

Nevertheless, student nurses should be encouraged to develop some of the skills involved within the research process, for example, those of information retrieval. A literature search and review is a good practical activity, enabling students to familiarise themselves with information retrieval systems. The teaching of such skills could be a joint initiative between teachers, researchers and librarians and could be addressed at the beginning of the course.

Each topic within the course should be linked with current research in the field in order to demonstrate the basis for the teaching and then applied to health care where appropriate. Research sessions, unless linked specifically to aspects of methodology should not be facilitated in isolation from other topics.

When students are on placements in institutional and non-institutional settings, they should be observing practice and questioning the rationale behind the care given in that particular environment. Unfortunately, this can create problems for some of the students as the qualified nursing staff do not always understand the motivation behind the questions and indeed cannot always answer the questions. It is at this stage where students can become disillusioned because they begin to experience problems of the theory–practice gap. This outlines the need to ensure that the professional development of mentors, in terms of nursing research, is most important; mentors should be facilitating learning.

The liaison teacher role could be utilised to support nurse practitioners in terms of demonstrating the use of research findings at the level of clients. If research findings are not being utilised in the areas where students are placed, then this should be addressed by educational audit and consideration given as to whether or not the placement is suitable for students (or indeed clients). Attempts should be made to help improve the situation rather than condemn it.

How should the level of achievement in research awareness be assessed?

The aimed level of achievement should be determined by the level of outcomes articulated in the curriculum. This will be at diploma level, and should be associated with the achievement of higher level cognitive skills, as measured against a model of competence such as that of Bloom. The higher level skills are those of analysis, synthesis, application and evaluation and can, in terms of research awareness, be demonstrated through levels of competence articulated within the assessment strategy.

As the student progresses through the course, weighting should be assigned to components of the assessment strategy and the further into the course the student goes, the higher the waiting should be for the levels of application, analysis, synthesis and evaluation (see Table 10.1).

Table 10.1: Possible weighting for theoretical assessment (percentage marks)

	Year 1 First assignment %	Year 3 Final assignment %
Knowledge	50	10
Comprehension	40	20
Application	10	25
Analysis	0	25
Synthesis/evaluation	0	20

The assessed course work should include assignments that will demonstrate an acceptable level of competence in research awareness. For example, components that would achieve this may include the literature search and review, essays related to practice, small scale studies of health care in a variety of settings and a research critique, linked to an aspect of health care. Such assignments are not explicitly related to research methodology, but encompass the necessary components, particularly when research has been an integral component in the teaching of all topics.

What should the level of research awareness achievement be for student nurses?

The acceptable level of competence is at the level of application, analysis, synthesis and evaluation decided and agreed within the assessment strategy, where is has been demonstrated that theory has been linked to practice, where students can read, understand and critically evaluate a research report and articulate its implications in terms of increasing the body of knowledge, changing policy or practice there-by contributing to the provision of high quality health care.

The health care media is constantly promoting the use of research findings in the delivery of client care. Health care professionals are constantly expected to make decisions about the ways in which client care is organised and delivered. These decisions need to be fully informed in order to promote and maintain quality in health care and the use of appropriate and relevant research findings can lead not only to excellence in care, but also to the intelligent and expedient utilisation of resources.

The time has come to develop a realistic and not too ambitious strategy for the promotion of nursing research. The profession should be addressing such issues as:

- *Raising awareness to research*
  At all levels.

- *Training in research methodology*
  A co-ordinated professional development programme based on need and incorporating quality monitoring mechanisms to prevent too many poor quality and inappropriate research projects. This programme needs to be flexible and affordable.

- *Improving education/service liaison*
  The only way forward in order to identify training needs, to decrease the theory–practice gap and to strengthen the basis for practice is by aiming research projects at

identifiable problems. Also to provide a teacher/practitioner support network in training areas, thus enhancing the learning environment for students.

The way forward is in educating student nurses in the theory and practice of research and attempting to remove the myth and mystery of a topic that needs to be perceived as an integral component of health care and not as a means to an end in terms of personal development.

References

Bell F (1984). *Patient Lifting Devices in Hospitals*, Croom Helm, London

Bloom B (1956). Taxonomy of educational objectives: the classification of educational goals, *Handbook One: Cognitive Domain*, David McKay, New York

Crosby C (1989). Method in mouth care, *Nurs Times*, **85**, 35, 38–41

David J A, Chapman R G, Chapman E J and Lockett B (1983). *An investigation of the current methods used in nursing for the care of patients with established pressure sores*, Nursing Practice Research Unit, Northwick Park Hospital and Clinical Research Centre, Harrow

Department of Health (1990). *Health Equipment Information No 98 (revised 1990): Management of Equipment*, Department of Health, London

Department of Health (1991). *Research for Health: a Research and Development Strategy for the NHS*, Department of Health, London, p 6

Department of Health (1992). *The Health of the Nation: a strategy for health in England*, HMSO, London

English National Board for Nursing, Midwifery and Health Visiting (ENB) (1992a). *Framework for Continuing Professional Education and Higher Award*, ENB, London

ENB (1992b). Additional Guidelines for the Development of Pre-registration Courses Leading to Parts 12–15 of the Professional Register and the DipHE, *Circular 1992/09/RLV*, ENB, London

Hughes J (1990). Stress, scourge or stimulant, *Nurs Standard*, **5**, 4, 33–50

Newcastle-upon-Tyne College of Nursing and Health Studies (1990). *The Clinical Liaison Standard, Curriculum for RN/Dip/HE*

1990 (unpublished), Newcastle-upon-Tyne College of Nursing and Health Studies

Nursing Times (1992). Research Nurse Advertisement, *Nurs Times*, **88**, 39, 115

Simmons B P (1983). CDC guideline for hospital environment control, *Amer J Infection Control*, **11**, 97–115

Thomas K (1984). Nomothetic, idiographic and hermeneutic social psychology, D307, Social psychology: development, experience and behaviour in a social world, *Metablock*, **8**, 109–111

Van Maanen J M (1979). From practice-directed vocation to research-based profession, *J Adv Nurs*, **4**, 1, 87–89

World Health Organisation (1978). *European Series 4*, World Health Organisation Regional Publications, Newcastle upon Tyne

11 Midwifery research
A phenomenological approach
Jeanne Siddiqui

This chapter adopts a particular application to midwifery research but the phenomenological perspective that is debated relates well to research practice within health care research. Furthermore, it identifies shared values and principles that underpin related curriculum, forms of knowledge and ethical considerations within nursing, midwifery and research practice generally.

Historical perspective

Promoting midwifery as a research-based profession has been beset with problems. Despite the introduction of research into the educational curricula, and creative efforts to infuse enthusiasm for research, there remains a theory/practice deficit. No matter how much education or information is given about research, there still seems to be a scarcity of midwifery research projects. More significantly, this indicates a continuing problem regarding the transfer of knowledge about research into the practice setting.

The statutory body for nursing, midwifery and health visiting, the English National Board (ENB) has encouraged the pursuit of *'the nature of knowledge that informs all practice'* (1989); others suggest that to resist the introduction of research consititutes neglect of responsibility which *'could be classified as professional negligence'* (Macfarlane 1984).

This attitude is reminiscent of cracking the proverbial nut with a sledgehammer. Rather than complain of midwives' obstinate refusal to become involved in research, those proselytisers of 'scientific enquiry' should first examine why midwives should undertake enquiry which will, for the most part, be unreflective of the nature of midwifery knowledge.

Hughes (1971) outlines how, in the past, the midwives' role has been artificially 'extended' as a result of research which encourages doctors to delegate to midwives tasks such as the siting of intravenous infusions, 'topping-up' epidurals and regulating the dosage of syntocinon. Sleep (1992) argues that 'these newly acquired skills do not represent midwifery innovations, prompted by the needs of normally labouring women'. Sleep's further remarks state:

> *'This well conducted trial (Prendeville et al 1988) has been reported in considerable detail; the paper includes the researchers' honest criticism of the trial design and conduct'.*

Surely, it is a fundamental duty of practitioners, doctors as well as midwives, to question and criticise and not to blindly accept that which either supports or nullifies their own views just because it is presented as scientific. In recent years, this emphasis towards the scientific mode of enquiry perpetuates the notion that the cognitive element of practice is more highly regarded than the psycho-social. Midwifery, however, is a social science and for research to be effective, it should be applied to practice and, at the same time, should effectively reflect practice as viewed by its recipients. Controversially, following her earlier remarks, Sleep goes on to say that we must question assumptions and challenge cherished beliefs about the effects of care. We are asked to consider accepting scientific enquiry as an efficient framework within which to *'protect families from the unintended adverse consequences of authoritarian prescriptions and proscriptions in perinatal care and education'* (Chalmers 1983). This statement, in itself, is one of the most dangerous and patronising attitudes which damages the reputation of research and which will make midwives resist even more strongly, the 'scientific' mode of enquiry. There must continue to be concern about any research method that views people as 'subjects', uses methodologies which are not easily transferable into the clinical situation and measures outcomes in statistical rather than human terms.

The concern for empirical reassurance in the area of professional practice stems from the influence of medicine in midwifery and the authoritative body of knowledge purported by doctors (Siddiqui 1992).

It is no accident that the isidious erosion of the midwifery profession has occurred during a period of history that incorporated vast social changes. Following World War II, the health of the surviving population came under close scrutiny. A benevolent government introduce the National Health System and was supported by the mutual paternalistic ideology of the medical profession. This ideology in turn, supported the rule-making and rule-following philosophy of a 'new' culture that challenged behaviour and experience in a commitment to 'social responsibility'. According to Stainton Rogers (1991), this caused a paradoxical situation because, at the same time, there was a commitment to self-expression and self-actualisation:

> '*On the one hand emergent feminist, Marxist, politically radical and civil rights groups were questioning what they saw as the 'psychology of the "good guys"' dominating theorisation in a way that portrayed women, ethnic minorities and the poor as 'deviant', and which failed to recognise the effects of inequality and disadvantage. On the other hand, the humanistic and self-actualization movements were questioning the mechanistic aspects of behaviourism that portrayed people as passive and mindless, denying individual creativity and spiritual values' (pp5–6).*

It was in this climate of social paradox in 1972, that the Department of Health and Social Security published its report on domiciliary midwifery and maternity bed needs, (Peel Report, HMSO).

Since the 1950s, hospitals had been promoted as the safest places in which to have a baby. The Peel report enforced this view with statistics that related to merinatal mortality, and which concluded by recommending that all births should take place in a consultant unit.

These findings, which have been authoritatively challenged and discredited over the years (Tew 1990), have caused long-lasting social and cultural effect, and significantly contributed to the undermining of the midwifery profession and the subordination of women by male doctors in an area of female supremacy.

Previously, midwives were independent practitioners who attended mothers in their homes (in 1930, 76% of babies were delivered at home); their standard of work was 'ruled by their own personal professionalism, apart from those sometimes bureaucratic local supervising authorities' (Cowell and Wainwright 1981). The isolation of the midwife and the rise in the birth rate led to a shortfall in the number of student midwives recruited to the profession. This shortage was overcome by trained nurses entering the field of midwifery practice and bringing with them a subscription to the medical model of care and the 'doctor knows best' philosophy.

A major outcome of these changes within the midwifery profession has been the increasing amount of intervention in the process of childbirth, directly related to the hospitalisation of pregnant women.

Tew (1990) questions the intentions of interventions which are *'devised by experts drawing on a wealth of scientific knowledge, to improve the ease and safety of childbirth'*. Tew asks if there are scientific reasons why they should fail in their purpose.

The facts are, that despite scientific research and a convincing argument from doctors, there are sound biological reasons why any intervention in the process of labour increases the risk of further intervention (Inch 1981), and is an inherent threat to the health and safety of mother and baby.

The medicalization of childbirth has been viewed by the feminist movement as a 'take-over' of women by men, yet women, themselves, have been and remain acquiescent in the face of this take-over. Andrea Dworkin (cited in Ethics – a feminist reader (1992), states:

> *'The conundrum of some women's willing and committed acceptance of policies and practices that condemn them to a*

restricted and inferior status is a central issue that feminism must face'.

Current perspective

Today, women are dissatisfied with the 'medicalisation of childbirth' (Carter and Duriez 1986). As a result of pressure from women and midwives, changes were introduced in hospital which attempted to humanise birth. However, Romito (1986) highlighted the fact that these changes were apparent rather than real, '*the changes do not challenge the power relationships between the expert and the childbearing woman*'.

Because the concept of childbirth is so linked to the psycho-social as well as the physiological processes, it is indefinable in the empirical sense. Attempts to measure its outcomes in these terms are usually deemed unscientific. If the empiricists are to make any sense of the process, it must be confined within measurable limits. Midwives must beware of this assumption that scientific enquiry is superior. This method of enquiry often focuses upon the 'product' or outcome with little regard for the 'process'. Dewey (1960) sums up the impact of viewing people in scientific isolation:

> '*The development of scientific enquiry is immature; it has not as yet, got beyond the physical and physiological aspects of human concers, interests and subject matters. In consequence, it has partial and exaggerated effects. The institutional conditions into which it enters, and which undermine its human consequences have not, as yet, been subjected to systematic inquiry worthy of being designated scientific.*'

It may be that midwifery and obstetrics have many fundamental ismilarities, not least the welfare of the mother and baby. The key element in midwifery research, however, must reflect the central focus of respect for persons. Features of the person, such as reason, self-reflection, morality, unity of mind and the active acquisition of knowledge rests upon a Kantian theory of the inter-relatedness of the 'knower' and the 'known'. Underpinning these concepts are the different assumptions that there is a phenomenal distinction between the mental and the physical processes, and nowhere is this more apparent than in the process of childbirth, where high levels of sensory stimulation affect the reaction and action of both the carer and the recipient of care.

If midwives are to be considered 'with woman', they must approach research through this perspective. In other words, through the phenomenological methods of enquiry. This may place midwifery in direct conflict with the scientific or objective outlook of obstetric research.

Phenomenology

It is said that science depends upon objectivity, measurability and formalisation, and as such, it seeks to reduce human nature to *'universal laws of action, experience and thought'* (Gergen 1986, cited in Stainton Rogers). This approach denies that individuals are able to manipulate, organise and constitute the world according to their own perception or consciousness. Yet the 'impersonal', 'objective' rules of scientific procedures and arguments are just as rooted in consciousness as any other forms of knowledge (Anderson p84).

Stainton Rogers in 'Explaining Health and Illness' is scathing about the 'obsession' psychology has with science, and proposes:

> *'....in assuming that researchers are sufficiently immune from the processes about which they are theorising, that they can sit in judgement about the meanings and purposes of others, their formulations are somewhat empirically limited'.*

Anderson endorses these views:

> *'When behaviourists and non-behaviourist psychologists alike, sought to achieve formality, objectivity, replicability and all the rest (sic), they so distorted their subject matter as to make their 'findings' irrelevant. The identities which are*

presumed between say, social conformity in daily life and social conformity in a Milgram experiment, or human learning and the acquisition of habit by rats are simply the result of a failure to reflect upon what their experimentation produces. Such reflection and clarification can only be brought about through a phenomenological sensitivity'.

Midwives cannot distance themselves from the subjective, emotive and spiritual nature of caring. To do so would be to deny the uniqueness and individualty of each person and their experience.

Benner (1984) points out that nursing (and by implication midwifery):

' *is rational and therefore, cannot be adequately described by strategies that leave out content, context and function....To assume that it is possible to capture* all *the steps in nursing practice is to assume that nursing is procedural rather than holistic'.*

The phenomenological approach seeks to examine the 'essence' of man in his world. John Paul Sartre, novelist and philosopher, referred throughout his literary work to the analysis of consciousness — the essence of man. He maintained that we are all in a process of 'becoming'.

'The taking of choices and the construction of being in our lives is the exercise of freedom and responsibility'.

In other words, man makes his own history (cited in Anderson).

Midwives are predominantly female, functioning as women, experiencing childbirth, child rearing and managing a family in the same way as their clients. This should mean that midwives are able to view pregnant women from a commonsense perspective. The basis of this view may be subjective but, if the argument that all knowledge (including empirical knowledge) begins in the consciousness holds true, then this same consciousness is subjective. What science does is to ignore the philosophical questions and, in so doing, ignores the human aspect of consciousness.

Phenomenologial research and philosophy

It is doubtful if there is an element of midwifery care that can be characterised as purely cognitive. Aspects may be rooted in a physiological foundation such as the process of labour. We may say that y will follow x in this process. This argument is only supported when there is absolutely no intrusion from the external world or anything within it. Similarly, the internal psychological processes, which are largely unexplored, may exert a particular influence upon the process in each individual. We can only say, therefore, that y will follow x if we can restrain ourselves from manipulating or interfering with the process. Heidegger (1967) suggests that this sort of attitude should be a case of 'looking on' without further concerns (unumsichtiges Nur-hinsehen – Being and Time, German ed). This stance maintains that we must deliberately desist from changing or interfering in what is before us. According to Immanuel Kant, 1724–1804, 'objective' or scientific knowledge is a form of idealism (Kant termed it 'transcendental idealism) which is based upon

■ how objects appear to us (phenomena), and

■ how they are in themselves (noumena)

Kant proposes that because our experience of the world is so mediated by our concepts (ideas), we can never have direct knowledge of things in themselves. All we can ever gain is knowledge through appearances. When dealing with the behaviour of human beings, it is dangerous to make generalisations based on the conclusions drawn from our observation of one person. All beings are individual; they undergo internal processes (thought, rationalisations, codifying etc) as well as external processes (reflex, response, behaviour).

It must be recognised, therefore, that any investigation which involves the behaviour of human beings must include how the person perceives his/her 'being' in the world. The notion of philosophical enquiry is particularly relevant in this context, for we cannot begin to examine people in their world without addressing issues related to concepts such as the use of language and the acquisition or 'nature' of knowledge. For example, midwives have often noticed how women's expectations of childbirth are influenced by what they were told by others, usually their mother. The language used by the mother, in particular relating to abstract concepts such as pain, will influence how her daughter perceives the pain of labour.

Philosophers have frequently asked how we come by the concepts or 'ideas' we have. The consensus view is that all the ideas we have or will ever have, come from our experience of the world as we perceive it. This experience evolves through the external senses, involving the physical world and from the inner senses, such as feelings of love, pain, pleasure etc. If it is true that all our concepts are derived from these two kinds of experience, then midwives must explore the concepts of childbirth with some confidence as women.

When trying to understand a concept, it is easy to fall into the trap of generalisation or of thinking that one construct of a concept is the same as another. It may be thought that a person must have a direct experience in order to understand a concpet. This cannot always be demonstrated, as the experience itself depends upon perception and the ability to express that perception in a language which has the same meaning for all. The use of language, however, does not stand alone; it is intelligible only within the context in which it is used and how it is viewed by individuals making sense of the world around them. The language used by midwives, pregnant women and obstetricians will be interpreted by each other according to the individual's life experiences, frame of reference and source of knowledge.

Each woman experiences childbirth in a unique way. The physiological process may be the same as many other women, and it is this process which may be viewed by the 'scientist' as representative of the broad sample. Having observed the physiological process, it may be said that the observer may have a 'concept' of labour. If this concept was a true and concrete picture of what every woman would experience, there would be no difficulty in advising women what to expect in the process of labour. One of the most commonly expressed emotions from women following childbirth, is that no-one told them what it was 'really like'. This is substantiated by Bradley, Brewin and Duncan (1983) who highlighted discrepancies between midwives' and women's perceptions of labour. It is only by exploring the sense-experiences of women during childbirth that midwives will be able to identify needs. The semantic meaning of the word 'labour' denotes hard work, and whilst childbirth is surely this, the word labour is too simplistic to completely portray the abstract meaning of the experience.

> *The act of childbirth has no adjective which can perfectly describe the feelings and emotions which occur in each individual woman at the time of the experience.*

It is through this understanding or admission that we begin to see how an acceptance of the limitations of our own experience must ensure that we keep an open mind on the subject of women's experience of childbirth. Midwives must use their knowledge and experience with the understanding that it is based upon perception. Midwifery knowledge must reflect the consciousness of 'being'. When we acknowledge this, we must also note that, when the source of our knowledge is based upon sense perception and experience, the conclusions we draw from the experience must include **deductive reasoning**.

In order to demonstrate how the midwife uses deductive reasoning in conjunction with her knowledge, and based upon sense experience, let us examine a familiar scenario:

1   The mother is experiencing painful uterine contractions

2   Contractions are necessary in order to expel the fetus

3   Therefore, the woman is in labour.

The premise (first statement) is an occurant state, experienced by the mother, whilst the inference (second statement) is based upon the midwife's experience. The conclusion (third statement) would have been arrived at using knowledge gained through experience, not only of the external sense perception but, equally, through the internal senses and the dispositional state of the midwife (essence of being).

The midwife's knowledge, together with the mother's behaviour, physical position, breathing pattern and the reported pain perception leads the midwife to the conclusion through the process of deductive reasoning. If we use this same scenario but examine it using empirical or scientific criteria, the conclusion may be different with serious implications for the mother.

1.   The mother is experiencing painful uterine contractions

2.   Contractions must be accompanied by cervical dilatation

3.   If cervical dilatation is not occurring, the mother is not in labour.

This is a well known obstetric viewpoint (O'Driscol *et al* 1975). Many women will present with uterine contractions, causing considerable pain and requiring alleviation of this pain. Because the empirical criteria is not met, they may be diagnosed as 'not in active labour'. The argument may be **valid** but this does not necessarily mean it is **true**. The conclusion follows logically from the premises but is **invalid** because phenomenological data such as time and space are not incorporated in the statements. Whilst it may be true that **eventually** the cervix must dilate, the occurant state of labour without cervical dilatation may also be true.

Application of phenomenology in midwifery research

We need to examine all research approaches when we are enquiring into the concerns of mothers and midwives. Most importantly, research which is qualitative and reflective of practice must be accorded equal prestige in the professional fields with that given to quantitative methods. Henry and

Pashley (1990) propose that central to qualitative enquiry is the phenomenological notion of how the individual person interacts in a world of everyday commonsense experience. This approach attempts to understand the meaning of experience through understanding the person's own perception and interpretation of the experience. Mischler (1979) confirms that the phenomenological approach 'does not seek one truth for the purposes of explanation but recognises that many different truths may be appropriate'.

One of the concerns that has puzzled the midwifery profession for a number of years has been the reluctance of mothers to breastfeed their babies. Many studies highlight that the inconsistency in advice given to mothers by midwives, may be responsible for the failure to sustain breastfeeding beyond the first few weeks.

There is an assumption that midwives, given the knowledge that breastfeeding is the best for the baby, should promote breastfeeding. It is true that many midwives do promote breastfeeding, but it is also true that many consistently project an attitude that is in direct opposition to the philosophy of breastfeeding. How many midwives and mothers have been asked what they think about the process? It may be that the questions to be asked should be about the perceptions of breastfeeding in a society which views the breasts as sexual appendages.

This is just one example of the necessity of exploring the perceptions of women, whether midwives or mothers, before we come to conclusions and make recommendations.

Henry and Pashley (1990) sum up the benefits of the phenomenological approac:

> *'It is appropriate to subscribe to the quantitative, scientific approach when the aim of the research is to measure particular variables, specific biological/physical aspects of individuals/institutions or groups, or to discover various statistical information, for example the number, age range and marital status of women undergoing caesarean section. A qualitative, phenomenological approach is more*

appropriate for subjective data that cannot be measured or clearly observed; it requires inference, assessment, reflection, interpretation and emphasis on meaning and understanding.

Individual differences in attitudes and conceptions cannot be adequately reflected through numbers; it is essential to take into account the meaning and use of language, and the subjective experience of the individual and their unique ways of perceiving'.

Conclusion

The future of midwifery research is dependent upon the appropriateness of the research tools used to investigate issues that are central to the concerns of mothers and midwives. These concerns have been reflected in the Health Committee Second Report on Maternity Services (1992). In the recommendations from this committee, the following extract should become the focus of all who care for women and their babies during a time in their lives which will provide them with a unique experience. The perception of that experience will remain with them forever. It may be that the only time they have the opportunity to report the perception of that experience is to their own daughter, influencing the perceptions of the next generation.

> *That the woman having a baby should be seen as the focus of care; and that the professionals prividing that care should identify their needs and develop arrangements to meet them which are based on full and equal co-operation between all those charged with her care. (Winterton Report 384).*

References

Anderson R J, Hughes J A and Sharrock W W (1986). *Philosophy and the Human Sciences*, Croom Helm, London, pp83–100.

Benner P (1984). *From Novice to Expert – excellence and power in clinical nursing practice*, Addison-Wesley Nursing Division, California.

Bradley C, Brewin C R and Duncan S L B (1983). Perceptions of labour; discrepancies between midwives' and patients' ratings, *Brit J Obstet Gyn*, **90**, 12 1176–1179.

Carter J and Duriez J (1986). *With Child – Birth through the ages*, Mainstream Publishing, Edinburgh.

Chalmers I (1983). Scientific enquiry and authoritarianism in perinatal care and education, *Birth*, **10** (3).

Cowell B and Wainwright D (1981). *Behind the Blue Door – The history of the Royal College of Midwives 1881–1981*, Bailliere Tindall, London.

Dewey J (1960). *Reconstruction in Philosophy*, Beacon Press, Boston pxxv.

DHSS (1970). Domiciliary midwifery and maternity bed needs, *Peel Report*, HMSO, London

Dworkin A (1983). Politics of Institutions, in Frazer E, Hornsby J and Lovibond S (eds), *Ethics: A Feminist Reader*, Blackwell, Oxford, pp100-131.

English National Board for Nursing Midwifery and Health Visiting (1991). *Guidelines for Midwifery Programmes of Education*, ENB, London. (Course leading to admission to Part 10 of the Professional Register – Registered Midwife (Eighteen Months)).

Heidegger C (1967). *Being and Time*, transl Macquermi J and Robinson, Blackwell Oxford.

Health Committee (1992). *Health Committee Second Report (Winterton) Maternity Services, Vol 1*, Feb, HMSO, London.

Henry C and Pashley G (1990). *Health and Nursing Studies for Diploma and Undergraduate Students: Health Care Research*, Quay Publishing, Lancaster, pp4–7.

Hughes E C (1971). *The Socialogical Eye*, Aldine Press, Chicago.

Inch S (1981). *Birthrights*, Hutchinson, London, Appendix 5.

Macfarlane J (1984). Foreword, in Cormack D ed, *The Research Process in Nursing*, Blackwell Scientific, Oxford

Mischler E (1979). Meaning in context: is there any other kind? *Harvard Educ Rev*, **49**, 119.

O'Driscol K, Carroll C and Coughlan M (1975). Selective induction of labour, *Br Med J*, 2 727–9.

Prendeville W J, Harding J E, Elbourne and D R Stirrat G M (1988). the Bristol Third Stage Trial: active versus physiological management of third stage of labour, *Br Med J*, **297**, 1295–1300.

Romito P (1986). The Humanizing of Childbirth: the response of the medical institutions to women's demand for change, *Midwifery*, **2**, 3, 135–140.

Siddiqui J (1992). Midwifery: Science or art? *J Adv Health Nurs Care*, **1**, 5, 3–12.

Sleep J (1992). Research and the practice of midwifery, *J Adv Nurs* **1992**, 17, 1465–1471.

Stainton Rogers W (1991). *Explaining Health and Illness – an exploration of Diversity*, Harvester Wheatsheaf, London, pp5–6.

Tew M (1990). *Safer Childbirth – a critical history of Maternity Care*, Chapman and Hall, London.

12 Research design and ethics

Glenys Pashley

This chapter specifically examines the aspects of good ethical practice involved in designing research. It is essential to clarify the research process, identifying in particular, the ethical value placed upon a 'good guide' or map. This chapter explores and attempts to synthesise important processes and levels taken to ensure the research project implicitly follows ethical guidelines.

Ethical issues are implicit within the research process. A major ethical concern in research practice, particularly for health care researchers, is a requirement to preserve the rights of the individual and, at the same time, generate knowledge.

Knowledge derived from the process of research is usually in the form of predictions, descriptions, explanations or it enhances our understanding of events. The form which the knowledge takes is very much dependent upon the level of objectivity, subjectivity and interpretation required and this is necessarily influenced by the nature and content of the subject under study. For example, quantitative research involves the researcher controlling the situation, manipulating the variables and collecting objective measurements, say, temperature, pulse and the depth and rate of respirations. Qualitative research utilises methods that place more emphasis upon subjectivity and the meaning of experience for the individual.

Whether the research is quantitatively based or qualitatively grounded, ethical issues are implicit, for instance, the duties and obligations of the researcher, the problems of control, manipulation, subjectivity and interpretation.

Therefore, it is essential for any researcher to construct the research design as a guideline for the research process. The major components of research design can be categorised under a number of headings:

■ identifying and clearly defining the research problem

- reviewing the literature in order to support the need for the problem to be researched
- the development of a conceptual framework
- identifying and selecting the appropriate research methods needed to collect the information for studying the problem
- processing, analysing and interpreting the information so as to determine a possible solution to the problem
- communicating the findings and recommendations

Inherent in this process ought to be the incorporation of an ethical framework which addresses such issues as: respect for persons; the rights of individuals, informed consent, confidentiality and responsibility. These and other ethical concepts are discussed in the light of each of the major components of the research design process.

Identifying and clearly defining the research problem

All of us are researchers in an informal way through our common sense knowledge, assumptions and questioning nature. During our lifetime we all experience particular problems that we would like to solve. Such problems may be personal, practical collective or intellectual. The process of research is a more formal way of pursuing solutions to our problems. According to Archbold (1986), the purpose of research is to seek answers to questions and to share the answers with others. This formal process involves activities of investigation, identification and analysis in order to either provide some answers to the questions or add to our knowledge and understanding of the problem.

As a starting point for any piece of research it is useful to ask some questions:

- What is the problem?

■ Who are the subjects for this research and how should they be selected?

■ What kinds of research methods will yield information that will help to solve the problem?

■ How can these research methods be refined in order to match the needs of this particular problem?

■ Are there any ethical implications which need to be considered?

A problem to be solved or researched could be, **'Is it really in the interests of some mentally ill patients to receive electro-convulsive therapy (ETC) as part of their treatment?'** As it stands this stated problem is too broad and general. For it to be researchable it needs to be more specific, particularly in terms of who the subjects are. It may not be feasible to ask some mentally ill patients what they think about their treatment. So, do we need to identify particular 'types' of mentally ill patients and would the hospital's ethical committee allow patients to be asked such questions? Perhaps it might be more realistic to ask the health professionals who care for those patients receiving ETC what they think. So, are we going to ask psychiatric nurses and/or doctors? The question, therefore, might more realistically be rephrased so as to read, **'What attitudes do psychiatric nurses involved in the administration of electro-convulsive therapy hold about this type of treatment?'**

Having narrowed the problem down to psychiatric nurses, we must then ask how they should be selected, how many should be included in the research, how much experience they should have and how we can obtain information about their attitudes (these issues of sampling and appropriate research methods are addressed shortly).

Once the question is posed it is possible to explore theories and previous research that might shed light on the problem. It is essential that research is not necessarily repeated. This emphasises the importance of reviewing the literature in order to support the need for the problem to be researched. However, prior to considering this second major component of research design, it is useful to discuss some of the ethical issues implicit prior to and within the research process.

The process of research generates many ethical issues. In response several professional organisations have developed guidelines and codes of practice (e.g. the British Psychological Society (BPS) and the Royal College of Nursing (RCN)). Such guidelines and codes embody similar principles which focus on the role of and competence of the researcher, justification for the study and issues related to informed consent, confidentiality, respect for persons, autonomy and the interpretation and publication of research findings. Particularly relevant to this first major component of research design are: the role of and competence of the researcher; justification for the study; and respect for persons.

The role and competence of the researcher and justification for the study

Self criticism and a continuous process of ethical analysis is central to the responsibilities of the researcher. He/she should examine what is right and wrong, evaluate personal values, beliefs and objectives, be conversant with guidelines and codes of practice and be prepared for potential role conflicts. Conflicting values can occur at different stages of the research process and often involve ethical and political issues, such as the decision to research or not to research, the nature of the questions to be researched and the problems associated with findings that may be detrimental.

The researcher will often experience multiple loyalties and obligations to those funding the research, colleagues, the subjects involved in the research and society in general. In this sense, the researcher must accept responsibility and professional accountability for the relevance and validity of the study under investigation. The researcher also has a duty to acknowledge the complexity of the research and so avoid trivialising and reducing complex issues to simplistic solutions.

A poor and unsound approach to what is a potentially complex research problem is not defensible on ethical grounds. Indeed, such an approach is more likely to do harm because it will produce irrelevant information and generate an attitude amongst colleagues and society that such researchers are perhaps incompetent.

Respect for persons

In carrying out any kind of research involving people, it is essential that persons are treated with respect. Respect for persons entails treating each person as an end rather than a means to an end. Also inherent to respect for persons are the terms: informed consent; confidentiality; privacy; rights; freedom and autonomy (cf chapters 7, 8 and 13).

Reviewing the literature in order to support the need for the problem to be solved

This second stage in the research design process is crucial in helping to identify and clearly define the research problems. In this sense, these first two stages need to be thought about in conjunction with each other. A research problem or an original idea tends to emerge from one's existing knowledge and experience to date, but such ideas can be developed more effectively from a review of what other researchers and theorists have discovered and written about directly and indirectly related problems and ideas. For this reason it is essential that the potential researcher broadens his/her knowledge base in order to compare and contrast what and how others have approached a similar problem. This broad and general review of texts and journals facilitates the researcher in formulating research questions or hypotheses that focus down on the problem in a more specific and precise way. In effect, the boundaries of the research problem can be clearly stated.

The ethical implications to be borne in mind here again concern the researcher him/herself. It is important that a critical stance is adopted to previous research findings, for example, other researchers' choice of methodology ought not to be easily accepted as the appropriate way to collect data but should be challenged and alternatives sought. Similarly, the researcher should not be afraid to challenge either the recommendations made by previous research findings or the theoretical framework upon which the study is based.

The development of a conceptual framework

A conceptual framework is a process that links the research problem and the underlying theory and which also ensures the formulation of clearly stated researchable questions or hypotheses that inform the methodology.

Table 12.1: Example of a conceptual framework

research problem	Why do some health professionals have a traditional view of the concept of persons?
theory	Philosophical theory from Aristotle to Wiggenstein/Psychological – Cognitive learning theories phenomenological perspective
concepts	'persons' deontological (spoken or written) rational language/meaning/use forms of life experience cognition learning styles concept formation
research questions or hypothesis	in their conception of persons, nurses and doctors are more likely to be influenced by the type of professional education they receive.

The area still to be clarified and which is central when deciding upon the appropriate methodology requires that the following criteria needs to be given some consideration:

■ sample of respondents

■ age range (mean age)

■ male and/or female

■ white/ethnic origin

■ nationality

■ social class

Having considered all of the possible variables that may influence the research it is then possible to address the choice of methodology.

Methodology

The types of methodology chosen to yield the kind of information required to help solve the research problem will be influenced by a number of factors:

■ whether the research contains elements of description and/or explanation and/or exploration

■ whether the research is quantitatively based or qualitatively grounded

■ how much time, money and resources are available

■ whether the research is to focus upon individuals, groups or social artefacts such as hospital data

Considerations about methodology bring to the fore numerous ethical issues which need to be addressed by the researcher, for instance, the subject's right to privacy, to be free from risk and harm, to be fully informed before consenting to participate or not in the research, confidentiality and autonomy.

Autonomy and informed consent

In relation to research the concept of autonomy implies that a person voluntarily decides to participate on the basis of information that increases their awareness and understanding of possible risks and benefits.

However, some forms of research, particularly qualitative research, does not always make it possible to offer the participant total information about the nature of the research, the methodology and the possible risks and benefits. For example, the use of an unstructured interview can lead to a discussion of issues not anticipated or unexpected events can occur involving the researcher and/or participants that can result in a modification to the research, thus changing the nature of the research to which the participant initially agreed. Since the researcher is sometimes unable to inform participants of the precise pathways involved in the research, informed consent might be better understood as 'informed participants', i.e. an ongoing process of information giving a possible exchange for continued consent and participation.

It is possible when informing participants completely of the nature of the research that the validity of the study is affected. Researchers are therefore placed in a position of sometimes having to deceive or misdirect participants. Smith (1975) argues:

> *It is generally recognised that deception or concealment is often necessary for research to be done validly because subjects may acts as they think the researcher wishes them to act.*

In cases where violation of informed consent occurs, one must ask, 'are the consequences to the individual outweighed by the consequences to the profession or society?'

Free from risk or harm

The researcher needs to be sensitive to what constitutes risk and harm. However, it is sometimes difficult to identify and generalise the levels of risk and harm because what is risky or harmful to one person may not be so for another person. Nevertheless, instances of risk and harm can occur and one typical example can be the use of the interview as a research method. The interview process, aiming to collect personal accounts of a respondent's life in order to understand his/her experience can be an intrusive technique that generates potential harm for the individual.

Privacy, confidentiality and anonymity

In research where the persons are the main source of information the principle of non-maleficence demands adherence to anonymity. Research can violate a person's privacy or result in labels being attached to a person which, in turn, might be used against the person in a harmful way. All attempts must be made to preserve the person's privacy, confidentiality and anonymity. However, the nature of the research cannot always ensure confidentiality, especially in a small piece of research where several people in the same organisation are respondents. As Archbold (1986) remarks, 'in small social systems where everyone knows everyone else, even slight clues... may reveal a person's identity.' The absolute right to privacy must be challenged. If the research reveals individual or organisational malpractice, then the researcher is placed in a position of having to decide whether or not to disclosed such findings (see next section for a discussion of this issue).

Analysing, interpreting and communicating the findings

The publication of results is a final but essential step in the research design process and illustrates the researcher's duties to the participants, funding body, professional bodies and society in general. The researcher has a responsibility to publish as much of the findings as possible without causing deliberate harm. It is in the domain of published results where potential conflict may arise; the person's right to confidentiality versus the public's right to know. The requirement of honesty on the part of the researcher is crucial. However, Leino-Kilpi and Tumaala (1989) acknowledge the presence of distortion of findings because of a researcher's bias, evident in the emphasis placed upon selection, omission of certain details or false interpretations. Possible motives for such distortion may be the production of results which lead to the researcher gaining recognition, status and/or promotion.

Research findings ought to be presented as simply, accurately and honestly as possible. The presentation of findings that are not clear to others for critical analysis can lead to controversy and harm. The subjective element inherent in the research should be acknowledged, as should other areas requiring additional exploration. Further, the researcher must clarify at the outset of the study his/her freedom in relation to publishing the findings, for some funding bodies insist on vetting possible publications, thereby exerting some degree of external control. In some instances this can be positive because there are cases where publication of findings can do more harm than good. Questions must be raised, however, when the publication of research findings are vetoed; is it because those in control are threatened and acting only in their own interests?

References

Archbold P (1986). Ethical Issues in Qualitative Research, Chenitz W C and Swanson J M (eds), *From Practice to Grounded Theory: Qualitative Research in Nursing*, Addison-Wesley, Wokingham

Leino-Kilpi H (1989). Research ethics and nursing science: an empirical example, *J Adv Nurs*, **14**, 451–458.

Smith H W (1975). *Strategies of Social Research: The Methodological Imagination*, Prentice Hall, New Jersey.

13

Research
An administrator's view
Janine Drew

This short chapter attempts to give a first hand account of an administrator who became involved in 'in house' research within a large organisation. It reveals, from personal and practical experiences, how it is important to motivate and encourage ethical research practice as a part of the process, sharing accountability inter-professionally. A multidisciplinary team is emphasised, recognizing the need for avoiding exclusivity in attempting to improve the quality of health care provision.

The aim of this chapter is to identify how research can contribute to the management and administration of health care provision, to focus on the difficulties likely to be encountered by individuals undertaking research for the first time and to emphasise the benefits to be gained, both professionally and personally, from research work.

It sometimes seems that the pace of change for managers and administrators who work in any organisation is too rapid and confusing. How is it possible to maintain professional integrity and cope with ever-increasing workloads when, to coin a phrase, 'the goalposts keep moving'. The Health Service in particular has had its share of change and challenge over the years in all areas of its responsibility — patient care, medical and nursing practices, management and administrative processes. The Patient Charter and shift in emphasis towards trust and status and private health care are only the latest in a long line of changes and innovations. Whether any changes in policy and practice being implemented in health care provision will ultimately be successful is unknown; although one would hope that the discussions and debates surrounding policy and practice have been well-informed and will, therefore, be effective and beneficial. One thing is inevitable, that changes will occur and any situation which may threaten the familiar and the manageable is often perceived as a direct threat to an organisation, the individuals working within it and the customers served by it.

For managers and administrators alike, therefore, changes can at best be seen as challenging, if bewildering, and at worst psychologically damaging in the extreme. For most of those involved, there is a sense of disenfranchisement; a sense of powerlessness in the face of greater forces at local, regional and national level. For many, there is often a lack of understanding of the wider issues and external demands which shape health care provision and its management.

Yet, is it not possible for managers and administrators to play a major role in the development of their particular service which will ultimately lead to the development and enhancement of the health care professional overall? This is possible through the exploration of professional practice by applied and action research. However, it is not a route traditionally associated with staff in such positions, whose personal development has normally been routed through the study of various professional qualifications and in-house training packages. Whilst any education and training can only be of benefit, these traditional routes tend to teach 'what is', not necessarily 'what might be' and 'why it is' and this is where research comes into its own. From an ethical and professional standpoint, managers and administrators should be involved in 'in house' research, which must ultimately benefit health care delivery.

However, the question arises, why should managers and administrators involve themselves in research in the first place as, in spite of the ethical argument, it would appear to conflict with their traditional role? There are many who would baulk at the commitment, personal motivation and time required to undertake research-based work. There is, no doubt, a personal sacrifice to be made which will impinge on all aspects of a researcher's professional and personal life and the pressures and stress involved should not be underestimated. In addition, there is the traditional view that research is either an academic and theoretical exercise or purely the preserve of the scientist and technologist. How can a manager or administrator undertake meaningful research? An important point to be borne in mind is that many issues affecting health care provision involve people and real situations and, therefore, purely quantitative research or theoretical analysis is not necessarily appropriate here. The emphasis must be upon qualitative research which relates to those situations which directly affect people, whether it involves the management of staff, the administration of the service, patient care or medical and nursing practices.

Having raised some concerns in relation to research work, the benefits should now be stressed. The sense of disenfranchisement and helplessness felt by many individuals working in the Health Service can be alleviated to a great extent by their becoming active participants in the framework within which decisions are made. Managers and administrators can enhance their own understanding of the issues affecting the profession by carrying out action research and by applying an already extensive knowledge to specialised research-based projects or higher education postgraduate work. The commitment and motivation necessary to undertake research not only leads to a development of the individual in terms of the acquisition of knowledge, but has tremendous impact in terms of enhancing personal self esteem and assertiveness.

Applied, or action research, is all about doing, not just theorising. It has been noted that action research involves small scale intervention, involvement and participation in the real world and involves close examination of the effects of that intervention. In addition, one of the principle aims of action research is to improve practice (Cohen and Manion, 1985). It would seem appropriate, therefore, in the context of the Health Service, which is constantly changing in order to respond to government policy, development in health care provision, patient demands and medical and nursing practices, to utilise a form of research which seems tailor-made to address these issues.

At a less personal level, but of equal importance, is the extent to which managers and administrators can use research in order to utilise their extensive experience and expertise in the development of appropriate professional practice and in assessing and monitoring the impact of policies and practice in real situations.

No one person can be an expert on every issue, but individuals researching in their own area of expertise can add to the body of knowledge available to the profession. It is also inevitable that undertaking research work, which is a very different experience from traditional methods of learning, can open up new personal insight and perspective and expand the mind. The learning curve can be difficult to cope with, but is ultimately intensely satisfying on a personal and professional level.

There are specific issues where research can help to facilitate the role of managers and administrators. In addition to the development of ethical codes and guidelines of professional practice, research can help to identify ways in which the strategic changes necessary for the development of health care policy and enhancement of provision can be managed and implemented. Research into human resource management can identify new methods of communication and interpersonal skills to help individuals in organisations, such as the Health Service, function efficiently and effectively and cope with the difficulties of constant change and uncertainty. The development of these areas will help to generate an ethos of collaboration and participation within administrative and management departments. By enhancing professional practice in the management of the Health Service, the people on the receiving end of health care will receive a service founded on sound research and practice, rather than empty promises and window dressing. A recent in-house project, which carried out an audit of ethics and values in a large university, is an example of how an organisation, through research based on its own difficulties and requirements, can harness in-house expertise to effectively perpetrate change. The problems faced by higher education in terms of funding challenges, management and administration and the pressure imposed by external agencies are not dissimilar to the health service and the methods applied in the EVA Project can be applied to health organisations equally well (Henry *et al*, 1992).

However, becoming a researcher in the academic sense of the word, when one has only been familiar with the often rigid and bureaucratic processes and procedures associated with administration and management, can be daunting. There is sometimes a sense of inadequacy and frustration when confronted by unfamiliar terminology and this can be compounded by the fear of having to get it right first time, as happens when preparing reports and interpreting regulations, the usual diet of the administrator. However, these fears are largely unfounded as, although the broad aims and objectives of the research and a plan of action must be identified at the outset to ensure that it is relevant and appropriate, nothing is cast in stone. The research itself, as it progresses, may dictate that work develops into unexpected areas of study or may have to change as the methodology chosen is seen to be inappropriate.

Nor is the researcher expected to work in a vacuum. If the research is being undertaken as part of a postgraduate course in higher education, for example a BPhil, MPhil or PhD, the work of a researcher is normally overseen by a Director of Studies, someone with expertise in the subject being researched and with experience in supervision. These individuals care on a day-to-day contact point and are there to consult, to give an objective view, to help with general housekeeping issues and, above all, to be supportive and give direction. Often, there is a second supervisor who, whilst not in day-to-day contact, fulfils a similar role to the Director of Studies. If the research is undertaken as a specific project within an organisation, there is usually an individual who will oversee the project and who will also fulfil the role of the more traditional, academic based Director of Studies.

One of the more difficult methods of conducting research is by bringing together small team work on a specific project. The difficulties lie in recognising the processes of group dynamics and in building a cohesive team which will agree to work by consensus to a common aim, often within a tight timescale. The ability to achieve balance of expertise and skill is essential as each individual will bring their own area of strength and weakness, personal belief and expertise which have to recognised and taken on board by the team as a whole. In addition, the values of participation, collaboration and respect are ethical considerations which will underpin the work of such a group. Any effective team should ideally work through the creative cycle of forming, storming, norming and performing. However, reality often dictates that this cycle of events cannot be adhered to and the process often has to be subsumed within the production of the objective. This problem, together with the intensity of the work being undertaken, often within extremely tight deadlines, can take a heavy toll on the interpersonal relationships within the group and needs to be carefully handled. However, the experience of working in an effective team can be exhilarating. There is an intense personal and professional satisfaction in working in a team towards a common goal where individual perspectives and expertise are acknowledged and innovative ideas can be generated in a spirit of co-operation within a supportive environment.

It may be an obvious point to make, but one of the first problems to be encountered, when the issue to be researched has been identified, is how to research and where to begin. This poses the tricky question of methodologies, the definition of which can vary wildly depending on whether one is a systems analyst or accountant or academic. It is important for the researcher to understand what he or she understands by the term 'methodology' because it is inevitable that at some point during the research, or on presentation of the findings, that the methodology used will be queried or even criticised. Research can succeed or fail on the basis of its methodology. Methodologies for purpose of research are the means by which data is collected i.e. through the use of questionnaires, surveys, interviews, statistics etc and the cohort or type of groups the data is obtained from. Good research will involve more than one method of data collection and will 'triangulate' information from at least three major sources in order to validate the data.

However, each method of collecting data and the means of identifying data sources have their own problems (Valentine, 1982).

Questionnaires are necessarily fairly generalised and need to be constructed very carefully in order not to bias the response. It is important to match the questions being asked to the research, in order that the data obtained is relevant. The questions themselves must be phrased in such a way as not to present any particular perspective or bias. Is a simple 'yes' or 'no' enough, or should there be a sliding scale, which would then make analysis more complex? Then there is the problem of how to interpret the data; should this be done manually or by utilising one of the many off-the-shelf statistical software packages available — some of which are helpful, some of which merely help to make a complicated problem even more confusing? In addition, it should be borne in mind that the response level for questionnaires is notoriously low and at least one third of the target group must respond in order to validate the information obtained.

Interviews, too, are difficult as the researcher, as an interviewer, will need to identify a relevant interview protocol or series of questions and acquire the skill to conduct an objective interview, again without leading the interviewee or biasing the response by subjective or irrelevant comments or body language. Again, does one restrict the interview to a specific set of questions, with no deviation, or is it more appropriate to conduct as semi-structured, open-ended interview where the interviewee is encouraged to respond in a far more general and open way to a series of more general questions? Then there is a problem of analysis, interpreting the content of the interview in order to draw out relevant information and knowing which data to ignore, however interesting it might be. How should the information be recorded? Most interviewees will probably be reluctant to present their views, particularly in relation to their own organisation, and will perhaps feel threatened if they feel the information they give will be presented in such a way that they may be identified. Therefore, it is important to assure an interviewee at the outset that the interview is confidential and that any data obtained will be presented in such a way so that the individuals concerned cannot be identified. If one intends to record the interview, or reveal the contents to another source, the permission of the interviewee must be obtained, not only as a matter of courtesy, but in order to fulfil the ethical good practice of obtaining informed consent. It is also good practice to offer a copy of the transcript of the interview to the interviewee. The researcher also needs to be aware that what is being said is not always what the interviewer believes and a good working knowledge of the politics or culture of an organisation can, therefore, be very helpful (Henry *et al*, 1992).

All this may seem daunting to someone unfamiliar with the practice of research. However, the techniques are actually not so far removed from that of everyday work undertaken by the manager and administrator. Both review and analyse information obtained from a variety of sources in order to draw out relevant data for the presentation of accurate reports; both attend meetings and are familiar with the techniques of listening and interpreting others' views and perspectives. Undertaking research is largely a matter of utilising those skills in a different way and focusing in greater detail on one or two specific issues.

It has been said previously that administrators and managers can play a major role in the enhancement and development of the health profession through research. However, shifting the emphasis of this role to incorporate research may cause some antagonism and even professional jealousy amongst traditionalists. It may be perceived that managers and administrators are acting outside their normal remit and this in itself can be perceived as a challenge to the *status quo*. Research into professional practice may be seen as a threat to the known order and balance of power within the organisation and it is important that the researcher is not viewed in Orwellian terms as the 'thought police', brought in to catch out the unwary. Some members in an organisational hierarchy, with a vested interest in maintaining their position and status, may also feel uncomfortable with the notion of research. There may be a perception that research by others will somehow remove their power, which has previously been based on exclusivity of knowledge. In addition, as has been said previously, changes — whether good or bad — are disruptive by their very nature and one response to threat is to behave in an aggressive or unhelpful manner (Schein E H, 1980). Not everyone, of course, will react in this way, but the issues should not be ignored. Again, a manager or administrator familiar with the politics and personalities involved will have a distinct advantage and will be able to steer his/her research through dangerous reefs far more effectively.

The impact of research on the professional practice of administrators and managers working in the health profession, and all organisations, is far reaching. There is an increasing awareness of the need for 'quality' and 'customer care' throughout all organisations, not just within the health profession. The parameters within which quality and customer care are defined will vary, but whatever definition is used, the health profession has a responsibility to build quality and care, whether it be the *Patient's Charter* or *Total Quality Management*, on a firm bedrock of research. If the issues underpinning the profession and the management of the NHS are not fully understood by those who implement the varying policies and practices, then promises of quality and care become facades without real substance Strategic planning and monitoring of performance cannot be undertaken in any meaningful way and the everyday reality of working in the profession becomes a series of management crises.

Research, by its very nature, brings about greater understanding of often complex issues, supports developments in health care, enhances the quality of provision and helps to manage change more effectively. The very fact that an issue is being researched raises awareness precisely because it is being researched. These outcomes, coupled with the application of research to real situations, can only bring positive benefits to any organisation, the individuals working within it and its customers.

References

Cohen L and Manion L (1985). *Research Methods in Education* (2nd edn), Croom Helm, London

Henry I C and Pashley G (1991). *Health Care Research*, Quay Publishing, Lancaster

Henry I C, Drew J L, Anwar N, Campbell G and Benoit-Asselman D (1992). *Report of the Ethics and Values Audit*, University of Central Lancashire, Preston

Schein E H (1980). *Organisational Psychology*, Prentice Hall Inc, New Jersey

Valentine E (1982). *Conceptual Issues in Psychology*, George Allen & University of London, London

14   Conclusion: ethical debate

Health care research

Christine Henry and Norma Fryer

Children cannot be
brought up in jars.......p5, M Midgley

Ethics is concerned with the thought processes behind moral judgements based upon debate of what is good, right and just. It has been reiterated several times throughout the text that ethics is implicit within the research process. Furthermore, in any kind of applied research the central focus is upon 'respect for persons'. This concerns the welfare and respect for respondents wishes.

A perspective in health care research may involve looking at the professional role, attitudes and values of doctors, nurses, midwives, applied social scientists, chartered psychologists, managers and administrators. Professional ethics underpinning research involves a multidisciplinary synthesis, simply because we are concerned with good practice in research, professional treatment and **care**. Wilcox and Ebbs (1992) rightly remark that scholarly activity and its outcome is a communal affair. From this standpoint the researcher is held accountable for both the process and the outcomes. Can the researchers detach themselves from the results of the project? It is important to note that those in health or social professional fields who are involved in research must take responsibility for the moral issues throughout the research process.

Policy and Codes

Should there be public policy in relation to research practice? if so what form should it take, a set of guidelines or a code of practice or should it take the form of a law itself?

As Kennedy and Stone (1990) point out, the way in which we decide to make public policy on any medical or moral issue, and what form it may take is rather haphazard and unorganised. Often this can be shown through crisis situations which attract the attention of the press, and there have been many. What happens is that a viewpoint may be sought, usually by the press, from someone who could be classed as a specialist to comment, then nothing follows until the next crisis. The most obvious example in relation to research occurred just after the 2nd World War, when there was outrage in relation to the exposure of Nazi Germany carrying out experimental research on persons in the concentration camps. It was only this that raised awareness and a need for a code of research practice. However, there has not been general identification of objectives or clear policy statements for over 50 years. There has been some attempt to develop Local Research Ethics Committee but even these are, geographically, unevenly distributed. These Ethics Committees have been set up to monitor research proposals, safeguard patients and clients' wellbeing but there has been no recognition for a universally applicable code of practice in relation to research across all professions. A code assumes consensus of values both within professions and for the public. An attempt through research to identify in one higher education organisation a set of shared values to start the process was carried out as late as 1992 (cf EVA, 1992, (Ethics and Values Audit abbreviated to EVA. This was a research-based audit)). The aim, in part, behind the EVA was first to identify shared values of an organisation that had a common aim, and to develop high quality education and research. The organisation had members who were professionals, researchers, educators, managers and administrators. The aim in part was to identify shared values then look towards developing a Code of Practice that would serve all members of the organisation. The Code of Research Practice would be a specific part of such a universal organisational code.

However, codes of professional practice are usually exclusive to one profession. The question arises, particularly in relations to research, 'should this be the case?' Should we formulate some clear direction through research to lay the parameters down for a national accepted policy relating to research practice?

Funding

How do you prioritise research funding? There is a conflict between the need to carry out basic research which might lead to fundamental changes in our understanding of disease and prevention strategies, such as health education or better professional practice and intervention. Funding will always be limited and difficult choices have to be made between major research that contributes to 'cure' or 'care'. For example, how much funding ought to be given to 'curing AIDS', as opposed to caring for those persons who are affected? Both raise ethical issues. Ethical theories such as utilitarian or deontological approaches may help to make informed decisions but do not give answers, for example, should the individual be sacrificed for the 'common good' or should value and respect for the individual take absolute priority (cf chapter 6)?

Miles (1990) remarks that there is no firm indication for future policy, as yet, that relates to funding of teaching and research, particularly in government resource allocation. Research imposes fairly substantial costs on the hospital or the organisations of the community where it is carried out. This cost has not been recognised and funded by the NHS regardless of the claim that a general duty is to support research.

Management of resource allocation involves ethical practice, particularly in identifying priorities. Radical methods of resource allocation are not understood by managers let alone the health care professionals. As was seen in chapters 2, 3 and 13, managers and administrators ought to be involved in research themselves, especially if the research encourages awareness and identification of priority areas.

Research may claim first priority for academic staff, simply because it yields money, travel, visibility and recognition of work in appropriate referred journals. However, carrying out research purely for its own sake, or for improving one's own publication record, is not ethically sound. Closely related issues in the role of funding for research projects show abuse in prioritising and raises ethical issues in both professional medical/health areas and in higher education. In the higher education sector, individuals are often put under pressure to obtain external funding, enhancing the value placed on competition with other institutions. Likewise, in professional areas, large research contracts given by industry to the medical researcher to test out a particular drug could lead to falsification of data in order to please the funding body. Researchers cannot detach themselves from the outcomes of their projects. Respondents/subjects must not be viewed as units or objects and any research that is poorly designed or executed is in itself unethical.

An important aspect of a professional who is clearly involved in either his/her own research or a medical research project, must ask whether the interests of the researcher may be in conflict with the respect and concern for patients'/clients' wellbeing. To disregard a person's rights in any research practice involves contradicting the basic principle of equal respect and value for all persons.

Most persons who are receiving health care are in some sort of need and, therefore, vulnerable. Researchers may be in a position to exploit the patients'/clients' vulnerability.

Autonomy and rights

The health care researcher is in a potentially powerful position in his/her role of researcher, practitioner or manager. However, as Faulder (1985) states:

> *Knowledge, like love, grows upon the appetite it feeds. The more we know, the more we feel it is our right always to be informed and consulted. The right to choose between options,*

> *the right to make our own decisions in short, the right to be*
> *asked for our informed consent... is the natural expression*
> *of our increased **autonomy** in medical matters (p 51)!*

To what extent does the health care researcher recognise the autonomous right of patients/clients? We know that there are difficulties with English Law recognising the autonomous rights, so perhaps it is reasonable to first ask the question of the professionals and debate what we understand to be the concept of autonomy and its application in health care for research.

The concept of autonomy was introduced in the first chapter, however, it is necessary to consider what the concept means specifically for the recipient, i.e. the patient/client who may become the respondent/subject in health care research? It is important that any 'moral rights' shared by both the competent (i.e. client, fellow, professional or student) and the 'incompetent'(i.e. vulnerable, seriously ill patient) are given separate consideration. The examples for debate centre around patient/client autonomy and relate specifically to the role of the health care researcher. This will, therefore, reflect the position of authority and power that the health care researcher holds within the present health care system.

The principle of autonomy holds a value based on 'human rights' and such a concept itself needs to be understood.

Human rights found their origins from 18th century philosophers such as John Locke and David Hulme, who shared a fundamental principle that the 'rights of man' ethic was based upon an implicit rather than a formal act of consent (Faulder, 1985). This meant that rights were fundamental. However, many of the fundamental rights identified by philosophers such as Locke and Hulme have become more commonly recognised as principles or guidelines relating to 'human rights' (often not recognized globally).

Generally speaking, 'human rights' reflect a moral code of practice that is also fundamental in recognising 'respect for persons'. According to Harris (1991) respect for persons, encompass concern for a person's welfare and respect for the person's wishes.

Nevertheless, there are times when 'rights' have been taken away in order to protect others or for the protection of a person from whom the right has been withdrawn. The most obvious example is shown when the right to freedom is taken away from those who are involuntarily institutionalised either because of a criminal offence or because of severe mental illness and where a person may harm themselves and others.

A more positive reminder of recognising 'rights' closely linked to understanding what is meant by autonomy, is the specific issue of women's rights in health care, particularly in relation to how reproductive rights of women were recognised from both a moral and legal stance following the Abortion Act of 1967. The Act brought complex moral and legal dilemmas which continue to arouse debate and conflict for health care practitioners, but it remains a significant landmark for women's autonomy throughout history.

Autonomy is a principle that supports the belief that a 'person' is free to control his/her life. Ideally, the principle of autonomy reflects the notion that a person is self-determined responsible and capable of making informed choices.

Nevertheless, the principle of autonomy is held to be an ideal concept that we can only approximate towards (cf chapter 1). A 'person's' capacity for being autonomous is influenced greatly by physical, psychological, social/cultural and political factors. Harris remarks that defects of control, such as mental illness, and defects of reasoning, such as prejudices that we hold, emotional views to implausible facts, will undermine autonomy. Furthermore, according to Harris, defects of information such as being misinformed and defects of stability are also influential in impairing a person's autonomy.

Harris uses J S Mill's argument that self determination improves not with time, but with practice. So, what of the 'person' whose role has become that of the sick individual and who may be asked to give their consent to such a research project? As a patient it is clear that there is an inevitable shift from the potential for self determination and control to the position of interdependence on other agents, be they practitioners, researchers or both. It is through the appreciation of the concept 'respect for autonomy', as distinct from the concept of 'autonomy', that a 'patient' may be allowed to maintain a level of control during a period of ill health (Brazier, 1987). The moral stance on autonomy of the competent patient/client focuses mainly on the issue of informed consent.(see chapter 7). It clearly reflects what a patient or client needs, in order to make an autonomous choice about medical treatment whether to participate in medical or health care research. Without such consent, a person cannot be said to have made an 'informed decision'. Defining competence in the context of health care and the law is itself difficult. However, it implies that the patient/client is in full control of his/her faculties and is consciously not under the influence of any outside physical or psychological agent. The patient/client will be able to make a rational decision. According to Faulder a test for competence is measured by the person knowing that he/she is giving consent and understanding what is involved.

However, another significant issue involves appropriate and adequate disclosure of possible consequences of medical treatment or therapeutic research (e.g. side effects of drugs). It is important to note the distinction between therapeutic and non-therapeutic research. Therapeutic research assesses forms of care or treatment and health care researchers ought to evaluate treatment and care and reduce any risk or harm associated with specific intervention. However, the participants in the research process may gain directly from the therapeutic study.

Non-therapeutics research is generally concerned with looking at management or education of the professionals, attitudes or social influences. The participant in the research process may not gain directly from the study but the outcome may lead to better care in the future. Conflict arises surrounding consent and subsequently autonomy when some health care practitioners hold the view that some patients/clients may not wish to be informed of all possible risks. The dilemma is really not one of choice about how much information should be given, rather that of whether the patient wants the information in the first place. The question of autonomy also gives the patient/client a right not to want full disclosure of details (i.e. respect for their autonomy).

It is important to note that 'informed consent' may be central to the concept of autonomy and a moral right for participants within the research process, but it is not a legal right in English law.

In examining the autonomy of the incompetent patient/client, the issue of informed consent presents a very different dimension for both the practitioner and researcher. The term 'incompetence' (still not clearly defined) is commonly used in law, whereas others may refer to reduced capacity for autonomy or by those who do not share full personhood (Henry and Pashley, 1990). Where a patient's/client's autonomy is compromised, he/she becomes reliant on decisions being made based on judgement and opinion of others. The mentally handicapped, mentally ill patients experiencing transient or permanent unconsciousness and children under 16 are all classified in this way.

A child's level of competence perhaps serves as a general example since the imposed position of limited autonomy is based solely on the child's age. English law places decisions to be made for minors, i.e. children under the age of 16 years, on the basis that they are made in the best interest of the child. Can this be said from a moral standpoint in relation to the child being part of a research project? It is suffice to say that there are many situations by the courts where the consequences of a decision are considered not to be in the best interest of the child (e.g. the Gillick case). Minors can be viewed to make autonomous decisions and, thus, it may be the case in relation to research. However, with a very young child, parental consent must be sought. The parents ideally should act as the child's advocate.

There has been an explosive growth towards persons' rights over their own bodies. The days have gone when the initial consultation meant any subsequent decisions made on behalf of the patient/client was implicitly accepted on the basis of the paternalistic relationship that existed between patient and practitioner/researcher, particularly the doctor.

However, there remains limits to how a patient's/client's autonomy can be protected. Brazier remarks that 'informed consent' lies at the heart of many other difficult problems of medicine, law and ethics (Brazier, 1987,p 193) and the law may serve as an obstacle to the rights of persons incapacitated by clients. Hence, it is crucial that the practitioner who takes the role of researcher must not only understand the ideal concept of autonomy and respect for autonomy but recognise the importance of 'informed consent' in relation to research practice. The central concern for both treatment and research is 'respect for persons'.

Attempting to identify a universal principle, allows for, at least the potential for developing an ethical system or theme integrated in research practice, running parallel to professional practice. With 'respect for persons' go the attendant moral concepts of autonomy, rights, beneficence, justice and, obviously, pursuit of excellent delivery of 'care' within health research practice.

References

Brazier M (1987). Patient autonomy and content of treatment: the role of the law, *Legal Stud J*, **7**, 169.

Faulder C (1985). *Whose Body is it Anyway?* Virago Press, London

Harris J (1991). *The Value of Life*, Routledge and Kegan Paul, London

Henry I C, Drew J, Anwar N, Campbell G and Benoit-Asselman D (1992). *Report of the Ethics and Values Audit*, University of Central Lancashire, Preston

Henry I C and Pashley G (1990). *Health Ethics*, Quay Publishing, Lancaster

Kennedy I and Stone M (1990). Making public policy on medical moral issues, Byrne P ed, *Ethics and Law in Health Care and Research*, John Wiley, Chichester, pp81–105.

Midgley M (1991). *Wisdom, Information and Wonder: what is knowledge for?* Routledge, London.

Miles M (1990). Research allocation in the NHS, Byrne P ed, *Ethics and Law in Health Care and Research*, John Wiley & Sons, WHERE?

Wilcox J R and Ebbs E S L (1992). *The Leadership Compass, Ask Erock George*, Washington University, Washington

Index

for Professional Ethics   107
for teaching research   128–129

H

Helsinki Declaration   69
Hidden Agenda   27
Humanism   46, 112
Hypocratic Oath   74

I

Integrity   4   see Morals
Informed Consent 9, 56, 64–66,
   69, 70, 73–85, 94, 99–101,
   107, 162–163
Imperatives   61, 63
Intelligence
   artificial 95–96

K

Kant   61–63, 68, 88, 97, 102, 144,
   146

L

Labour
   in childbirth   148
Leadership
   training   18–23

M

Materialism   111
Measurement
   of data 114

Meritocracy   29
Methodology
   see Research
Morals/Morality
   awareness 60
   dilemmas 52, 57, 74, 78, 83
      99–100
   education 11
   integrity   8
   laws   5, 61–64
   professional code of   10
   responsibility   10
   values   9, 91, 106

N

Neuroscience   98
N.H.S. 16, 19, 21, 25, 28, 30–39,
   120, 141, 167, 169, 170, 175
Nurenberg Code see Codes
Nurse Researchers   123, 124
N.T.V.S.   National Vocational
Training Schemes 121

P

Paternalism   78–80, 84, 100, 141,   185
Pathology 108
Patient's Charter see Charter
Peel Report   141
Phenomenology 112–113,   144–151
Placebos   44, 83, 84
Positivism 45, 97, 111–114
Psychology   45–47
   see Applied Psychology
Public Sector 32–36
Principles
   of Autonomy, see Autonomy
   of Research, see Research